SUGAR CRUSH

SUGAR CRUSH

How to Reduce Inflammation,

Reverse Nerve Damage, and

Reclaim Good Health

DR. RICHARD P. JACOBY

AND RAQUEL BALDELOMAR

HARPER WAVE

An Imprint of HarperCollins*Publishers*

This book contains advice and information relating to health care. It is not intended to replace medical advice and should be used to supplement rather than replace regular care by your doctor. It is recommended that you seek your physician's advice before embarking on any medical program or treatment. All efforts have been made to assure the accuracy of the information contained in this book as of the date of publication. The publisher and the author disclaim liability for any medical outcomes that may occur as a result of applying the methods suggested in this book.

HarperCollins books may be purchased for educational, business, or sales promotional use. For information, please e-mail the Special Markets Department at SPsales@harpercollins.com.

FIRST EDITION

Designed by Fritz Metsch

Library of Congress Cataloging-in-Publication Data

Jacoby, Richard (Physician)
Sugar crush : how to reduce inflammation, reverse nerve damage, and reclaim good health / Dr. Richard Jacoby and Raquel Baldelomar.
pages cm
ISBN 978-0-06-234820-3
1.Sugar—Health aspects. 2. Sugars in human nutrition.
3. Inflammation—Prevention. 4. Nerves, Peripheral—Diseases—Prevention. I. Baldelomar, Raquel. II. Title.
QP702.S8J33 2015
612.1'2—dc23 2014048822

15 16 17 18 19 OV/RRD 10 9 8 7 6 5 4 3 2 1

CONTENTS

PART III: SO NOW WHAT'S STOPPING YOU?

—————

I t is exciting to be at the tip of the spear in the war on sugar.
It is a war that not only we United States citizens have
been losing; it's also being lost by anyone in the world who
eats prepared food. Only farmers still living off the land and
eating the fruits of their own labors are safe.

Sugar, *sweetie*, and *honey* are terms of endearment, but
not when we consume sugar to the extent that it has become
responsible for more deaths per year than the Vietnam War,
more deaths per year than alcohol, and more deaths per year
than tobacco.

I personally first became familiar with the effects of
sugar as a child, during my early visits to the dentist. Ouch!
The memories border on post-traumatic stress. The re-
maining deposits of silver in my teeth are testimony to the
insidious destruction of our bodies by sugar. In my adult
life, there is the continual struggle to keep myself from becoming prediabetic or even diabetic. You can only exercise

so much, and then you must take control of your own diet. This is where this exciting new book, *Sugar Crush*, enters the picture.

Dr. Richard Jacoby, coauthor of *Sugar Crush*, has been my friend for more than a decade, since the first time I met him in my Advanced Lower Extremity Peripheral Nerve Workshop. He was already an expert foot and ankle surgeon. He responded to my lectures and teachings about the relationship of the peripheral nerve to sugar and to chronic nerve compression in a way the other 352 students of my thirty workshops had not. Perhaps it was his background in chemistry. Perhaps it was just simply his ability to incorporate my surgical research related to chronic nerve compression, my basic science research related to diabetes and chronic nerve compression, and his own patients' relief of pain and recovery of sensation in those who responded to the surgery he learned to do in that workshop. Rick Jacoby has now moved well beyond the operating room.

Sugar Crush is an intriguing detective story implicating the food industry, processed foods, marketing, well-meaning but misguided nutritional science, and an individual's "Bliss Point" for carbohydrates in a conspiracy that places sugar at the crime scene of many of our most common diseases and disabilities.

My own life has already improved since reading *Sugar Crush*. I was able, having been educated now by my student, to go through the prepared foods in my own kitchen cabinets and discard those with lots of sugar; replacing them with healthier yet still tasty substitutes.

While the food industry will not like the information contained in *Sugar Crush*, I believe readers interested in improving their own health, and the health of their families, will treasure this book and use it as a road map to improved health.

A. Lee Dellon, M.D., Ph.D.
Professor of Plastic Surgery
Professor of Neurosurgery
Johns Hopkins University

INTRODUCTION

—————

*All truth passes through three stages. First, it is ridiculed.
Second, it is violently opposed. Third, it is accepted as
being self-evident.*
—ARTHUR SCHOPENHAUER

The Why Should I Read This Book? Quiz

(Check Each Truthful Statement)

☐ When someone serves birthday cake, I like the piece with the most icing.

☐ There's a supersized jar of Excedrin in my office desk drawer.

☐ I've had a medical procedure with the suffix -*ectomy*.

☐ I could lose a few pounds, but I don't need another diet book. They don't work.

☑ Sometimes at night, my feet itch or feel tingly.

☐ Every winter I have a runny nose; every spring I get sinus headaches.

☐ I *love* anything crunchy/salty and can drink olive juice straight from the jar.

☑ I'm often tired. In fact, I could take a nap right now.

☐ My parents and/or grandparents had diabetes.

☑ I like my toes and want to keep them.

SCORING:

1 to 2 items checked: Let's consider denial.

3 to 4 items checked: Not bad, but you should read on.

5 to 10 items checked: Forget about the weight you'll lose; this book could save your life.

So What's the Book About?

My purpose is to get your attention—to demand you recognize how *sugar*:

- chemically causes inflammation that damages your nerves,
- results in excruciating pain often made worse by prescription drugs, and
- will inevitably kill you before your genetic timetable.

Carbohydrates (sugar) + Trauma =
Nerve Damage, Pain, and Dysfunction

This is the sugar crush. And it begins with subtle clues such as having too many headaches, a runny nose, adult acne, and a diet full of salty snacks, chocolate, and processed foods.

I'm asking you to derail the express train taking you straight from sugar to peripheral neuropathy—then onward to diabetes, cardiovascular disease, stroke, and many other neurologic disorders—including multiple sclerosis (MS), migraine, carpal tunnel syndrome, and Alzheimer's disease, to name a few.

Why a Podiatrist?

Peripheral neuropathy is the clarion call I witness every day. And it's noisy. It's what literally wakes you from your sleep. It is painful. Like hot needles, it stings and it burns. It starts in the autonomic nervous system of your legs and feet, then on to the sensory fibers, and finally lodges in the motor fibers.* That's usually when I'm called in.

As a young surgical student in Philadelphia, I experienced my first amputation—to remove a gangrenous leg from a man suffering with diabetes. Even though I'd spend the next thirty years as a podiatric surgeon and conduct tens of thousands of foot surgeries, including amputations on patients with diabetes, this first gruesome procedure is the one I remember most.

I was the third assistant. My job was to hold the rotting leg as the orthopedic surgeon sawed it off just above the knee. The stench of a gangrenous leg is putrid and overpowering, so much so that we had to put peppermint oil in our masks to endure it. As I held the leg and struggled with the smell and the sound of the saw, I was struck not only by the impersonal, awful nature of the procedure—but by the enormous weight of the diseased leg as it fell into my arms.

I stood confused in the middle of the room. Clutching the heavy burden and wondering what to do with it, I saw a nurse nod toward the medical waste container. No longer viable, this once healthy, functioning leg was now trash.

That amputation was the end result of diabetic peripheral

---

*Nerves in the peripheral nervous system (all else besides the brain and spinal cord) signal your body to, first, feel and then move.

neuropathy—precipitated by pain and numbness, caused by damage to the nerves of the foot. Had we not removed this man's grossly infected leg, the gangrene would have killed him. But how did it get to that point? This is the question that eventually led me to write *Sugar Crush*.

There's no reason for you to wait until someone like me must cut off your gangrenous toes or relieve the pressure of your inflamed nerves, when the answer could be so simple.

Stop eating sugar.

Richard P. Jacoby, D.P.M.
Diplomate, American Board of Podiatric Surgery

PART I

This Fine Sweet Mess

1

The 500-Pound Canary

A SUGAR TSUNAMI

Regardless of metaphor, we should address the painfully obvious. Each year, the average American eats 160 pounds of processed sugar.

And by sugar, I mean all of the -*ose* and -*itol* words: glucose, fructose, dextrose, sorbitol, polyglycitol, galactose, and others. It's difficult to find out just how many "chemically sugar" compounds are approved by the U.S. Food and Drug Administration (FDA) for use in food, toothpaste, vitamins, or nighttime cold medicines—but it's more than simply being labeled "sugar." And that's not counting consumption of alcohol. Pervasive seems too weak a word. We love sugar; a spoonful of it makes anything go down.

Meanwhile, 40–50 percent of American adults will develop diabetes (those at greatest risk are Hispanic men and women as well as non-Hispanic black women). Obesity is the main factor in the increase in diabetes among all demographics. The treatment and care of diagnosed patients cost approximately $174 billion per year. If you have diabetes, you're also two to four times more likely to experience a stroke. That means your brain stops acknowledging a major part of your body. Your arm, your legs. The side of your face. Oh, yeah, and your bodily functions falter. We haven't even gotten to cardiovascular challenges. Or breathing. But you get the picture.

Diabetes

Presently, most forms of diabetes are categorized in three groups:*

- type 1, in which the body's immune system destroys the cells making insulin
- type 2, in which an individual has too little insulin or cannot process insulin
- gestational, which can occur in pregnancy if a woman's hormones interfere with insulin production.

This book is concerned with type 2 diabetes and the primary culprits surrounding its causes, progression, and control.

As early as the 1990s, I saw a crisis developing around peripheral diabetic neuropathy, foot ulcers, and amputation—direct results of the increase in diabetes. The number of people being diagnosed with type 2 diabetes was skyrocketing—even kids were getting it. Remember, it's well understood that this chronic disease is directly linked to lifestyle. Combine a diet high in sugar (including fruits, honey, and starch—all of which

*There are surgically or chemically induced types of diabetes, as well as latent autoimmune diabetes, but those are the topics of other discussions.

turn into varying amounts of sugar when digested) with a lack of exercise and the eventual result will be type 2 diabetes and all the miserable complications that come with it.

The link between sugar and *diabetes mellitus type 2* is the defining trait of the disease. *Diabetes* comes from the Greek, meaning "siphon," as in siphoning water out of the body. *Mellitus* comes from the Greek word for "sweet." Put them together and what you have is a very descriptive term for a symptom of diabetes: sweet urine. And for thousands of years, physicians tasted a patient's urine—if sweet, the diagnosis was diabetes mellitus. Another way of diagnosing diabetes in the ancient era was to observe if a person's urine attracted bees. Today we're a little more sophisticated about it—we conduct blood tests to check your plasma glucose (blood sugar) level.

The Dinner Guest Who Just Moved In

Sucrose is the chemical name for refined or table sugar (be it white or brown, organic or packed with pesticides) and it consists of two carbohydrate molecules—glucose and fructose. But you don't get off that easily. Sucrose is also the primary component in fruit juice, milk, yogurt, honey, molasses, and maple syrup.* Until the early 1800s, refined sugar was still a relatively expensive product and most of us didn't eat that much of it. Jack Challem, a nutrition researcher and the author of *The Inflammation Syndrome*, calls refined sugar a genetically unfamiliar ingredient. He observes that "a lot of health problems today are the result of ancient genes bumping up against modern foods."

---

*More about all of these in Part III and the chapters on diet.

In the late 1700s, the discovery that crystallized sugar could be extracted from the sugar beet, along with increased sugarcane production in the tropical areas of the world, meant that the price of sugar dropped. Soon sugar was an everyday food, no longer a luxury product to be locked away in silver boxes.

At the beginning of the twentieth century, while sugar was a bigger part of the standard diet than it had ever been in human history—most people still ate only about 25 pounds of it in a year. Today, consumption has roughly quintupled. As I mentioned earlier, the average American now eats about 160 pounds of sugar every year, or slightly more than 7 ounces a day. To visualize this daily amount, imagine taking the teaspoon next to your morning coffee and filling it 27 times with sugar. In reality, much of that sugar enters our diet in the form of highly processed snack foods. In fact, the top eight sources for *half* of the average American's diet are: soft drinks, sweet baked goods (cake, doughnuts, etc.), pizza, salty snack foods (potato chips, corn chips, popcorn), bread products (bread, rolls, bagels, English muffins), beer, and French fries or other frozen potato products.

The link between sucrose and obesity, with its compounding symptoms of high blood pressure, high blood glucose, high cholesterol, as well as ancillary conditions such as migraine headaches, carpal tunnel syndrome, gallbladder disease, irritable bowel syndrome, reflux disease, and other chronic health issues, is irrefutable. Robert Lustig, pediatric endocrinologist and professor of clinical pediatrics at the University of California, San Francisco, simply calls sugar poison.

Even without an official diagnosis of diabetes, you could already be experiencing the earliest signs of neuropathy:

those little zings in your wrist; the occasional burning sensation in your feet; the mild numbness in your fingers that comes and goes; and the headaches that come out of the blue. These are all harbingers of things to come.

And yet, despite this rap sheet, sucrose has an even more destructive twin.

High-Fructose Corn Syrup

While regular sugar is about half glucose and half fructose, high-fructose corn syrup (HFCS), as the name suggests, is up to 55 percent fructose and only about 45 percent glucose. This matters because the more fructose, the sweeter the taste. However, the most insidious distinction comes because the fructose in both sugar and HFCS is more quickly converted to fat (metabolized and stored) in the liver, a precious organ that has plenty to do besides dealing with yet another toxin. Meanwhile, the glucose in both refined sugar and starchy carbohydrates can be metabolized by any cell in your body. Reading a book, running a marathon, breathing—any cell called to action uses the energy of glucose to keep you going.

We'll talk more about the metabolism of sucrose and HFCS (and how they most often turn into fat) later, but it can get confusing so, for now, a quick crib sheet:

- Carbohydrates contain the simple sugars sucrose, glucose, and fructose.*
- Sucrose (table sugar) is 50/50 fructose and glucose.
- HFCS has more fructose and tastes sweeter.
- Fructose quickly metabolizes in the liver (which has

---

*A fourth sugar, galactose, is found in dairy products.

enough to do already), often leading to what's known as a "fatty" liver.

- Glucose, on the other hand, can be metabolized by every cell in the body, meaning you have a better chance of burning it off.
- Ergo, fructose is a double whammy.

And yet, when this "sweeter than sweet" product first became available in the 1970s, it seemed a miracle, solving a huge problem in the American food supply. Because at that time, the cost of plain ol' sugar had risen sharply, primarily due to international trade tariffs and sugar quotas in the United States. Fun sweets and crunchy/salties were costing more. Maybe people could learn to do without them.

This new, inexpensive sweetener, made from corn grown in the United States (and subsidized by the government), was just what the food industry needed to keep order. In fact, high-fructose corn syrup turned out to be not only cheaper than sugar, but, from the perspective of industrial food producers, it was better.

The "sprinkles on the cupcake" was that it's also a liquid, and thus easier to combine with other ingredients, such as flour for hamburger buns and flavoring for soft drinks. That's why fast-food restaurants were suddenly able to offer their soft drinks in larger sizes for the same money—and why you sometimes get a free soda with your pizza delivery.

High-fructose corn syrup is one of the primary reasons that portion sizes—and waistlines—have ballooned in recent decades. Americans today consume the equivalent of 12 teaspoons a day of HFCS alone; that works out to be about 10 percent of our daily calories.

There's one additional consequence of the way high-fructose corn syrup has largely replaced sugar in our manufactured foods. Mercury contamination has been documented in a frighteningly high number of snack foods made with high-fructose corn syrup. Mercury-grade caustic soda (street name, lye) is a key ingredient in the complex milling process that separates the cornstarch from the corn kernel, the first step in creating HFCS.*

Secret Sugar

The food industry hides the added sugar in their products under a lot of different aliases, evil twins, you might say. But sugar is sugar. When you check the ingredients label, skip the product if any of these more common weasel words for sugar is among the first five ingredients:

Agave nectar
Barley malt
Beet sugar
Blackstrap molasses
Brown rice syrup
Brown sugar
Cane sugar
Caramel
Carob syrup
Coconut palm sugar
Corn sweetener
Corn syrup
Corn syrup solids
Crystalline fructose
Date sugar
Dehydrated cane juice
Dextrin
Dextrose
Dried oat syrup
Evaporated cane juice
Evaporated cane juice
 crystals

*Some researchers report organic mercury (methylmercury) being left behind in this process and ending up in food products made with HFCS. Mercury is a potent neurotoxin; no amount of it is safe because the body doesn't have an efficient way of getting rid of it. So it is possible that heavy consumers of junk food have also accumulated mercury that could be damaging their intestinal tracts, nerves, and kidneys.

Fruit juice concentrate

Glucose

Golden syrup

Gum syrup

High-fructose corn syrup

Honey

Inverted sugar

Malt syrup

Maltodextrin

Maltose

Maple syrup

Molasses

Muscavado

Palm sugar

Rapadura

Refiner's syrup

Simple syrup

Sorghum syrup

Sucanat

Sucrose

Treacle

Turbinado

And Let Us Not Forget Booze

Eat the bread with joy and drink the wine with a merry heart.
—ECCLESIASTES 9:7

Okay, sounds good. And yet, metabolically speaking, if sugar has an evil twin, then "drinking alcohol" *can become* the demon spawn. This is because sugar converted to booze converts to ethanol plus carbon dioxide, and if you imbibe—do not pass Go. Do not collect two hundred dollars. Go straight to the liver. It's all about intake volume.

How Your Body Copes with All That Sweetness

In order to recognize sugar's destructive powers, it helps to understand how your body reacts to it. As the British physiologist and nutritionist John Yudkin details in *Pure, White, and Deadly*, refined sugar is a substance for which your body has "no physiological requirement."

As mentioned earlier, when sugar enters your body, simple carbohydrates are quickly dismantled into glucose (which passes directly from your intestines into the bloodstream to be used for quick energy) and fructose (which moves through your liver to generally be stored as fat). So far, so good. Your body needs glucose to function efficiently (as in breathing or jaywalking), as well as some fat to store energy (for the lean times) and to cushion your organs.

But the human body has evolved to get limited sugar from naturally sweet sources such as vegetables and fruits in season (meaning not *everything* all year-round) and the occasional taste of honey—all of which release glucose and fructose into the bloodstream slowly. Nothing in your biologic history has prepared your body for the onslaught of concentrated sugar that you now pour into it every day.

As a result, glucose spikes. If energy needs are high at the time, sugar is efficiently put to good use and metabolized, which is to say that it is broken down to build up the components of cells. However, a sugar supply that's either too frequent or too heavy pushes your pancreas into overdrive, causing it to release excess *insulin*—the hormone that transports glucose into your cells to be burned as fuel. A squirt becomes a spew as insulin struggles to escort glucose into your cells by brute force.

After years of a poor diet, and being overweight and sedentary, your cells become more and more resistant to the mission of insulin. And if you're still packing in the sugar, your blood glucose continues to rise as your overworked pancreas simply wears out. You make less and less insulin as your cells become more and more resistant to it. That's called *insulin resistance*.

But before your pancreas gives up completely, all of that

excess insulin and blood glucose lead to inflammation—and
that's when the real trouble begins.

Sugar and Inflammation

So let's assume your body is flooded with sugar and HFCS.
A newly understood phenomenon, *inflammation*, underlies
modern health scourges, from heart disease to obesity to diabetes. "Sugar can play a role in inflammatory diseases," says
Dave Grotto, R.D., formerly a spokesperson for the American Dietetic Association. "Poor regulation of glucose and
insulin is a breeding ground for inflammation."

Under normal conditions, "acute" inflammation is a good
thing, helping you rebound from injury. For instance, if
you cut yourself shaving, white blood cells race to the scene
to mop up the wound, destroy bacteria, and mend tissue.
"Chronic inflammation" (also called low-grade or systemic
inflammation) is another matter.

Chronic inflammation:

- damages your immune system,
- can be painful,
- raises triglycerides, cholesterol, and blood pressure, thus
  contributing to diabetes and heart disease, and
- is implicated in conditions ranging from allergies, asthma,
  and inflammatory bowel disease to fatigue, depression,
  wrinkles, and dry skin.

(Carbohydrates)   **Chronic**
    Sugar   =   **Inflammation** + Trauma   =
        Nerve Damage, Pain, and Dysfunction

What Causes Chronic Inflammation?

While there are genetic causes, the most important factor is believed to be the standard American diet, rich in pro-inflammatory compounds (all those ugly carbs we just discussed) and lacking antioxidants* and other nutrients that help and control inflammation. A. Lee Dellon, M.D. Ph.D., professor of plastic surgery and neurosurgery at Johns Hopkins University School of Medicine, said, "When the injury is deep inside the body, such as inside the nerves servicing any end organ,† hidden inflammation can trigger pain, trauma, and chronic disease. Experts are only beginning to understand how sugar fans these flames."‡ John Cooke, M.D., with the Cardiovascular Laboratory at the Stanford School of Medicine, is a cardiologist by training, with an additional Ph.D. in vascular biology. He believes inflammatory substances like sugar cause the inner lining of arteries to become more like Velcro, rather than the normally smooth, Teflon-like surface.

But as you might well suspect, it gets worse.

---

*Essential nutrients found only in food (primarily vitamins C and E), antioxidants are the chief defense against the attack of *free radicals*—nasty by-products of the body turning food into fuel. They're called "free" because they're missing a molecule and in trying to bond with another molecule, they can damage DNA and cell membranes. Free radicals contribute to atherosclerosis, cancer, vision loss, and a host of other chronic conditions—including aging.

†The specialized receptor of a peripheral nerve—that is, heart, kidneys, gangrenous toe, eyes, etc.

‡By the way, acidity is yet another factor. Most Americans eat a generally acidic diet caused by too much salt, sugar, white flour, dairy, and cola drinks. Many experts consider overacidity to be one of the major causes of chronic inflammation.

2

The Nerve of It All

HOW CHRONIC INFLAMMATION CRASHES
YOUR MIRACULOUS HARD WIRING

*If the central cell body were the height of an average
man, its axon would be one or two inches in width
and would extend more than two miles.*
—THOMAS B. DUCKER, M.D.

B ite after bite, sip after sip, sugar is inflaming your blood
vessels and nerves. This unrelenting inflammation incites
stress in the body's natural repair system, which results in *fibrosis* (scarring). The ongoing scarring systematically, perva-
sively, and insidiously causes compression in any area where
blood vessels and nerves pass together through a tight area.
I call this the Global Compression Theory* and throughout
the rest of the book, we'll explore how and why this happens.
As well as what you can do about it.

---

*It would be easy for me to yield to medical convention and call this an
hypothesis—an educated guess based on observation and my experiences
as a surgeon—because in the medical paradigm, a *theory* is something that
can be disproven through clinical trials. And I challenge anyone to do so.
In the meantime, while you wait for medical bureaucracy to catch up, you
could simply cut sugar out of your diet and save yourself.

You Studied Nerve Cells in Middle School

Because this is a chapter about nerves, I first thought I should display detailed illustrations of various neurons—actual cells. Break it all down. Or tell you that such depictions always reminded me of a deep-sea creature or a scorpion, every detail serving a magnificent purpose: the cell body (*soma*) containing your DNA—with its tentacles (*dendrites*) that receive electrochemical messages; and the *axon*, a segmented tail-like appendage that whips those messages out to other cells in the body.

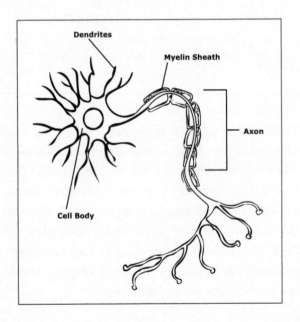

Yes, it is the cell that supports and nourishes the axon and its supporting (insulating) structure called the myelin, but it is the *interruption* of the proteins within this structure that causes the symptoms of end organ damage and eventual

death of the neuron itself. This concept is in contradistinc-
tion of neuron death by all other direct insults to the nerve
cell itself, for example, in trauma or when *poliomyelitis* destroys neurons through viral disease.

My concern here is to explore how inflammation and your
body's natural defenses lead to compression of the nerves
themselves. A good example is the wrist, where the *neurovascular bundle* (artery, vein, and nerve) passes through a
narrow, bony tunnel. Compression in this tight area leads to
the hand pain, tingling, and loss of sensation seen in carpal
tunnel syndrome. Any compression around a neurovascular
bundle in a *fibro-osseous tunnel** ends up restricting healthy
blood flow to the nerves. This leads to malfunction of whatever the neurovascular bundle connects to—the end organ. If
your nerves don't get a fresh blood flow, they're starved for
oxygen and other nutrients and their waste products don't
get efficiently carried away.

Think of it this way. Your nerves conduct electrical messages just as an electrical cord conducts electricity. Turn off
the power or dial back the dimmer switch and the lights
go out or begin to fade. That's what's happening with your
nerves. As your body struggles to deal with the inflammatory impact of sugar, your nerves become damaged, swollen,
and compressed as they pass through fibro-osseous tunnels
in your body. As they are compressed, they essentially begin
to flicker—like when insulation around an electrical wire gets
wet. The current no longer flows steadily and nerves become
less and less effective in carrying out their essential function
of relaying important messages from your brain to muscles

---

*When normal bone is replaced by fibrous connective tissue, further com-
promising these tight spaces. A perfect example is the dental demise requiring a root canal.

and organs throughout your body. Again, the ultimate result is damage to the end organs: the gangrenous toe, the blind eye, the damaged heart.

How Your Nerves Work

Imagine arriving at an ocean beach on a hot day. You cross blistering pavement in the parking lot and step onto the sand to remove your shoes and socks. Immediately you feel the raspy texture and unstable footing below as you walk across the hot, rough surface to find a nice, smooth spot to spread your beach blanket. Then down to the water, and as you go, your feet begin to cool even as you may also feel the occasional sharp or blunt edge of a seashell. You feel the changing texture of the sand, along with the cold water as it washes over your feet. All this time, you've been unconsciously balancing yourself to compensate for the changing surfaces—while sensing temperature, pressure, vibration, touch, and pain.

These sensations and that *proprioception* (knowing where you are in relationship to your environment) start with tiny cells in the skin on the soles of your feet. I'm going to focus here on the way you perceive sensations, not your whole nervous system (that would be another book). So, here we're talking about the nerves of your *afferent nervous system*—the ones that perceive sensations and send messages about them to your spinal cord and brain. I'm also going to focus just on the nerves that affect your feet, although pretty much everything I'll discuss also applies to the rest of your body.

Sending messages about touch, temperature, pressure, and pain starts just under the surface of your skin with several different types of receptors:

- Mechanical receptors sense stimulation by pressure, such as stepping on the sharp edge of a seashell.
- Thermal receptors sense temperature changes.
- Polymodal receptors sense unpleasant stimuli, such as pain.
- In skin that doesn't have hair, like the soles of your feet, you have two main kinds of mechanical receptors: *Merkel cells*, which sense changes in pressure, texture, and location, and *Meissner's corpuscles*, which sense light touch and vibration. You have two types of thermal receptors: one to detect cold and one to detect heat. Messages about pain also start just under the skin surface through tiny nerve endings called *nociceptors*.

All of this simply means that when a receptor senses something—when you step on a pebble, for instance—that mechanical message gets converted to an electrical impulse that's relayed up the line to your spinal cord and brain through nerve fibers. You feel the shape, size, and sharpness of the pebble underfoot because your nerves are relaying those important messages.

We're talking about feet here, but the part of your body with the most Merkel cells is your hand. In fact, that's what your fingerprints were designed for: Merkel cells cluster under the raised ridges. When you pick up a hot cup of coffee, Merkel cells are what make your fingers so exquisitely sensitive to touch and pressure. These important nerves are how you feel the shape and texture of the cup, which enables you to grasp it effectively. The Meissner corpuscles do the same for the perception of movement and vibration as the Merkel cells do for touch and pressure. Stop for a minute and pick up an object—a cup, a rock, a book, anything will do.

Close your eyes and think of all of the ways that you know what you are holding: the shape, the temperature, the texture, whether it's wet or dry, etc.

You have similar raised ridges on the soles of your feet.

In another analogy, Merkel receptors are like pixels. The more pixels your screen has, the clearer the picture. The more functioning Merkel receptors you have, the clearer your sensations of shape, texture, or pain. Long-term nerve damage from sugar destroys these receptors and as they die, the picture gets increasingly fuzzy. When your nerves can't adequately read the surface beneath your feet, all kinds of problems begin to arise. You lose your balance and you can't feel pain, so you don't necessarily know when you've hurt yourself.

Nerve Fibers

When axons bind together, they form *nerve fibers*. These structures come in several types as well, but we'll focus here on the two most important kinds: *type A delta fibers* and *type C fibers*.

Type A Delta Fibers

Type A delta fibers are sensory nerve fibers. They're myelinated, meaning they're wrapped in a thin layer of a fatty substance called *myelin*. For the A delta fiber, myelin acts much as insulation does on a wire carrying electricity. Myelinated nerves conduct sensory information quickly. When you step on something sharp and cut your foot, the A delta fibers send the message to your brain and you feel a sharp pain almost instantly. Likewise, if you dip your foot into the cold ocean, you feel the sensation of cold very quickly.

Type C Fibers

Type C fibers are also sensory nerve fibers, but they're un-myelinated and are much thinner than A fibers, and so they transmit sensory information more slowly. They also need a stronger stimulus to go into action. In general, C fibers are responsible for telling your brain about sensations such as burning pain, temperature, and itchiness. When you have a dull ache or chronic pain, your C fibers are relaying the message.

When you look at how tiny all these receptors and nerve fibers are, it's easy to see how too much sugar in your blood-stream can damage them. A Merkel cell is cup-shaped and only about 10 micrometers in diameter.* C fibers are only 0.2 to 1.5 micrometers in diameter. When very thin, unmy-elinated nerve fibers are constantly bombarded with excess glucose, they easily get *glycated*, or clogged up with oxidized glucose that sticks to them, just as caramel candy sticks to your teeth. The A delta nerve fibers are myelinated, so they get damaged when too much glucose makes them swell up and compresses them within the myelin sheath. Too much sugar can even make A delta fibers demyelinate and lose some of their fatty sheath.

And with every type of receptor and nerve fiber, excess sugar keeps the blood vessels that nourish them from ex-panding and contracting normally—the blood flow is uneven or even blocked, causing further damage. Eventually, when the nerves are damaged enough, they stop conducting, leav-ing you with permanent numbness.

When your sensory receptors aren't working well, you don't feel things properly. You might not notice that a fold in

---

*A micrometer is a millionth of a meter, or 0.000039 inch.

your sock is giving you a blister, for instance. Alternatively, the sensory receptors can become supersensitive and start overreacting to or even imagining sensations. That's when your feet might become very sensitive to heat or cold or you might feel as if you have a pebble in your shoe even though you don't.

And when your nerve fibers aren't transmitting messages up the line from the receptors very well, it's like a blurry picture, or static on the line. Some messages don't get through at all, causing areas of numbness. Other messages get distorted or amplified, causing pain, itching, and burning. If the larger A fibers have started to demyelinate, it's like having cracks in the insulation of an electrical wire—you get a short circuit that might even cause a fire. That's pretty much what happens to your nerves when they demyelinate.

More interesting, perhaps, is that when any of the afferent nerves are damaged, they don't need a signal from a sensory receptor to send a message. They can start firing off at random with the sharp, sudden pains that are so characteristic of diabetic peripheral neuropathy. They can also become hyperactive and extremely sensitive, sending a signal of severe pain from even the lightest touch. Some of my neuropathy patients can't stand the touch of even a bedsheet on their feet; others are supersensitive to heat or cold. Let's drill down even deeper into how all this happens.

Three Key Chemical Pathways

Over the years, all of that extra glucose has literally been gumming up your nerves through inflammation and scarring. Such inflammation occurs over three main pathways: the Maillard reaction, the polyol pathway, and the nitric oxide pathway.

The Maillard Reaction

The Maillard reaction is the *chemical interaction** between glucose and amino acids whose result we recognize in flavorful brown food, like corn roasted on a grill or what happens to turkey skin in a hot oven. Named after French chemist Louis-Camille Maillard, who first described it in 1912, the Maillard reaction also takes place in the human body, where it's called *glycation*. Glycation occurs when glucose in your system reacts with proteins, fats, or nucleic acids (DNA) to produce advanced glycation end products (aptly abbreviated AGEs). They're produced when a protein reacts with sugar, resulting in damaged, cross-linked proteins—causing them to become stiff and malformed. On your skin, this results in wrinkles and age spots. Imagine the same internal reaction throughout your body and you have an idea of what AGEs are doing to you.

AGEs are a toxic form of scar tissue—keeping the nerves from functioning properly and causing lesions. As the body tries to protect itself by breaking these AGEs apart, immune cells secrete large amounts of inflammatory chemicals. Many of the diseases we think of as a part of aging are actually caused by this process. Depending upon where the AGEs occur, the result can be arthritis, heart disease, cataracts, memory loss, wrinkled skin, or complications of diabetes—such as peripheral neuropathy. One way to look at it is that you're slowly cooking your nerves to death, just like that turkey in the oven.

---

*The process in which atoms rearrange themselves to form a new substance. In doing so, they either absorb or give off heat/energy.

The Polyol Pathway

When you have more glucose in your system than your body can use or store, your body has to get rid of it some other way. So it reverts to the fallback method: glucose is metabolized through a complex process called the *polyol pathway*. We don't need to go into all the details of the pathway, because the damage to your nerves happens right at the start, when the glucose gets broken down via an enzyme (or biological catalyst) called *aldose reductase* into a substance called *sorbitol*. Sound familiar? It should. Commercially derived from stone fruits, seaweed, and—you guessed it—corn, sorbitol is often labeled as an "organic sweetener" in low-cal processed foods, dietetic candy, and imitation crab, to name but a few.

Sorbitol cannot pass through cell membranes, which means that it gets stuck wherever it's made. And because sorbitol is chemically related to sugar, it attracts water. (Think of your sugar bowl on a humid day.) When sorbitol starts to build up inside a cell, it also draws in water, which makes that cell swell up. The swelling itself is bad, because it reduces blood flow to the nerve, starving it of nutrients and oxygen. But when the swelling occurs in places where the nerves pass through a tight tunnel, such as your wrist or ankle, there's not enough room. The nerve gets compressed within the tunnel, causing pain, numbness, and all the other symptoms of neuropathy.

The Maillard reaction and the polyol pathway are two processes that are well understood and well documented in the medical literature. There is nothing new or surprising about them. The next part, however, about the nitric oxide pathway, *is* new.

The Nitric Oxide Pathway

Your blood vessels have an inner lining called the *endothelium*. An essential amino acid in your blood, *L-arginine*, goes through a complex process involving the enzyme *nitric oxide synthase* (NOS) and converts into the gas *nitric oxide*. When the endothelium releases this gas, it causes your blood vessels to relax and your blood flows freely through the vessel.*

When the endothelium is damaged, it can't create nitric oxide as well, which means your blood vessels don't relax as they should. How does the endothelium get damaged? As with every other chemical reaction in your body, the answer is complex—but in this case, the molecule *asymmetric dimethylarginine* (ADMA) is an important factor.

Hang on, we're almost there.

An amino acid found naturally in your body, ADMA is structurally very similar to L-arginine. We could call them cousins. And so both ADMA and L-arginine can attach to the enzyme nitric oxide synthase (NOS).

When L-arginine attaches, it converts to nitric oxide and your vessels function the way they should. When ADMA attaches, however, it converts to *peroxynitrite*,† which clogs the conversion and blocks the production of nitric oxide. (Not good.) Technically speaking, ADMA inhibits nitric oxide synthesis. Too much ADMA in your blood (also linked to insulin resistance) causes your blood vessels to constrict rather than dilate.

---

*One reason why nitric acid supplements are all the rage.

†The chemical symbol for it is, rather appropriately, OONO.

You Can See Where I'm Going

Here's how I believe inflammation and scarring from sugar causes nerve damage:

1. Too much sugar triggers inflammation in your blood vessels and causes the Maillard reaction, or glycation: the slow-sugar-cooking of proteins in your body. Among other things, this makes the endothelium rough and sticky, rather than smooth. As Cooke noted, it becomes more like Velcro than Teflon.

2. When sugar is processed into sorbitol, it enters your nerves through the polyol pathway and gets stuck there. The sorbitol causes your nerves to absorb water and swell. When there's no room for them to expand further, the nerve gets compressed against the surrounding bone and tissue. The pressure causes pain and numbness. In addition, the swollen nerve gets less oxygen and nutrients as it gradually stops conducting effectively.

3. The nitric oxide pathway is blocked by high levels of asymmetric dimethylarginine (ADMA). This causes the blood vessels to constrict, which reduces blood flow to the nerve—and reduced blood flow means that the tiny blood vessels bringing nutrients and oxygen to your nerves constrict and then clog up.

A relatively minor amount of constriction can lead to a disproportionately large impact on flow. According to Poiseuille's law,* a 19 percent reduction in the radius of the vessel will reduce blood flow by 50 percent.

---

*A theory borrowed from fluid dynamics that helps describe the flow of blood through a vessel.

Think of the implications. Less than 20 percent constriction results in blood flow being cut in half. And when nutrient- and oxygen-rich blood can't get to your nerves, they suffocate and black out, slowly and painfully.

Back to Global Compression

The takeaway is that such mechanisms are at work everywhere in your body and account for such diverse problems as irritable bowel syndrome, migraines, and macular degeneration. To see the complete picture of what happens when you eat sugar, it's important to remember that your nerves are essential messengers throughout your body. They fulfill roles that extend well beyond the sense of touch, carrying critical messages to and from every muscle and organ in the body. When those messages are impaired, muscles don't work properly and organs fail. Even if you never experience an appendectomy, a similar story applies to the bodily mechanisms behind other end organ ailments. The nerves that control the large intestine, for example, can become damaged, and lead to the alternating diarrhea and constipation that are the most common symptoms of irritable bowel syndrome. Headaches are similar in that the occipital nerves controlling muscles in the head can become irritated and entrapped, just as the nerves controlling the gallbladder or the big toe in diabetic peripheral neuropathy.

All nerves are irritated by the effects of sugar and ultimately damage important muscles that control the functioning of your organs.

3

Killing You Softly

THE CREEP OF COMPRESSION

By the time you notice the symptoms of diabetic neuropathy from nerve compression in the tarsal tunnel of the foot, you've had uncontrolled high blood sugar for a very long time. You've probably experienced a series of ailments through your life that were actually unrecognized symptoms of sugar's slow, insidious damage, including Bell's palsy* or Morton's neuroma.† These seemingly unrelated events are actually signals from your body that sugar is taking a relentless toll on your health and that you're slowly moving down a path toward diabetes and death.

---

*A partial (and often temporary) paralysis caused by inflammation and compression of the seventh cranial nerve—a nerve traveling through a narrow, bony tunnel called the Fallopian canal.

†Patients often describe this common and painful thickening in the ball of the foot (most often between the third and fourth toes) as "walking on a pebble."

Type 2 diabetes confounded the medical community because it's a *conformational* disease—conformational meaning there's a misfolding of proteins.* One example is *kuru*,
a fast-acting conformational disease that comes from eating
a human brain already infected with a misfolded, infectious
protein. The incubation period can be decades, and when the
disease becomes active, a slow, agonizing death takes about
a year. Mad cow disease is a similar conformational disease
that has an incubation period of up to eight years and, like
kuru, kills slowly, over a long time.

I'm not suggesting you'd knowingly eat a human brain
or a mad cow. Even though both diseases are rare, it's important for our discussion that several scientists, including
Dr. Melvin Hayden, in the journal *Pancreas*, have identified
diabetes as also being a conformational disease of the pancreas.† Hayden notes that it may take up to forty years before
we appreciate the full effects of this process. In other words,
there's a long gestation period between cause and effect.

How the Steady March
to Diabetes Goes Unrecognized

Because a conformational disease such as diabetes can "mis-
fold" proteins slowly, it can be nearly impossible to discern
how, exactly, one thing leads to another. Most people who
have type 2 diabetes have been incrementally approaching

---

*Normally a protein "folds" and assumes a three-dimensional shape
needed for adequate functioning. A misfolding can occur for many reasons, including extremes of temperature or pH, as well as other chemical
and mechanical disruptions. "Misfolded" proteins not only don't work;
they can also have toxic qualities.

†And, yes, you're right—the pancreas does look like a brain.

that diagnosis for many years, even decades. The inexorable nerve damage from years of high blood sugar has been leaving clues and warning signs all along, although most doctors never connect those dots. Why?

First, doctors are highly trained in their specialties, which can prevent them from taking a step back and seeing the not-so-apparent links between one kind of "-itis" and any another. Second, even as a diet high in sugar and processed carbohydrates is doing its damage, by the numbers—that is, from your standard blood test results—your blood sugar may seem fine and not raise any red flags.

If doctors aren't trained to look for the linkages, they won't see them. In fact, diabetes isn't a disease that doctors typically detect or respond to until it's too late to turn the ship around. By the time a blood test gives confirmation, your blood sugar levels have been too high for far too long and the pancreas is too destroyed to undo the damaging effects.

The Revolutionary Decompression Procedure

As a traditionally trained podiatrist, board certified in foot and ankle surgery, I was treating diabetic wound infections the way I'd been trained, like every other doctor on the planet: medicine, surgery, or amputation. Again, I was treating the effect of the disease, not addressing the underlying cause. Sick care—not health care.

In the late 1990s, I started hearing about a remarkable surgical procedure for treating severely compressed nerves in the foot. It was developed by A. Lee Dellon, M.D., Ph.D., one of the leading peripheral nerve surgeons in the country and known for perfecting the technique of surgical decompression of peripheral nerves, including the median nerve at the wrist (carpal tunnel) and the ulnar nerve in the elbow. In this minimally invasive procedure, the surgeon makes a small incision in your skin. Then, instead of removing a swollen nerve, he or she relieves pressure (decompresses) by opening tight tunnels around the affected nerve. And so even if still swollen, the nerve returns to normal functioning. No more pain.

When it comes to operating on my patients I'm very conservative, and so even though I thought the Dellon procedure might have value, I was still skeptical. The results seemed too good to be true. When I studied his method, I couldn't find a controlled trial for it. Because I'd been taught that a controlled trial is the gold standard for evaluating the success of a new medical anything—drug, device, or surgery—I felt that this new approach wasn't ready for prime time. And certainly not for my patients.

Even so, I was intrigued. The Dellon procedure not only claimed to restore sensation in the foot, it seemed to keep further damage away. Moreover, after surgery, his patients didn't get seem to get any ulcerations or need amputations.

When Dr. Dellon was scheduled to speak in my home state, I was first on the sign-up list. Afterward, we had a chance to talk, and the conversation turned to the standard treatment for Morton's neuroma. He asked, "Why do you [podiatrists] cut nerves out of the feet?"

I was taken aback and found myself answering, "Because that's what we do."

In other words, I was simply following the standard procedure that I'd been taught, and without questioning if it made sense. But here was one of the leading peripheral nerve surgeons in the world asking me why we removed the nerve.

Mind you, it is the only nerve that is treated in that way—by simply removing it. It was a moment of recognition for me. I had to stop and ask myself, "Why *are* we removing this nerve?" His question was the catalyst that led me to rethink everything I knew about not only Morton's neuroma, but the nerves of the feet in general. Ultimately it led, almost in a straight line, to this book.

The Dellon Decompression Surgical Procedure

Dellon had first experimented with the effects of compression after reading an important paper by Drs. Adrian Upton and Alan McComas on carpal tunnel syndrome published in 1973 in *The Lancet*, a well-respected British medical journal. At that time, carpal tunnel syndrome was widely believed to be a mechanical problem brought on by repetitive motion, like typing on a typewriter. This repetitive motion led to inflammation, which "crushed" the *median* nerve in the carpal tunnel. However, Upton and McComas had made the interesting observation that 16 percent of the patients they studied with carpal tunnel syndrome also had diabetes. They suggested that diabetes was potentially causing a "second crush" on the nerve. Dellon saw that bit of data and wondered what it might mean. He did an experiment with rats to better understand what happens when you have a double crush.

Proving the Double Crush

First, Dellon put thin silicone tubes on the rats to compress the tarsal nerves on the distal end (away from the body, just above the foot). In other words, he created a single crush on the nerve bundles in the rats' feet. The rats showed no symptoms of neuropathy, and gait was not affected. He then added a second band closer to the center of the body, near where the extremity attaches to the torso (proximal). Immediately the rats began to show symptoms of neuropathy—staggering, wobbling, and unsteadiness when walking. Dellon extrapolated from the Upton and McComas observation and his own experiments with these rats that if you could surgically decompress the nerve in the carpal tunnel in humans (in other words, cut one of the bands to release the pressure), you could fix the crush, the symptoms would disappear, and function would return to the nerves. This led directly to the development of *decompression surgery* to relieve carpal tunnel syndrome. If you cut into the fibrous tissue compressing the swollen nerve and give the nerve room to expand within the tight fibro-osseous tunnel of the wrist, the symptoms disappear.

The Next Scientific Step Forward

Then in the late 1980s, a patient who'd had his carpal tunnel pain relieved with Dellon's new decompression procedure asked him, "You fixed my hands; why can't you fix my legs? I have the same pain there. Can't you do something?"

Dellon told his patient, "We don't do that," because that was how he'd been trained. It seems counterintuitive, but conventional medical thinking then was that nerve problems in the lower extremities (legs and feet) had nothing to do with nerve problems in upper extremities (elbows, wrists, hands).

He tried testing the idea with a new series of fascinating experiments. The goal was to see if compression in the lower extremity was, in fact, the same as compression in the upper extremity. He dipped the feet of normal, healthy rats in ink and had them walk across a piece of paper to study their gaits. Everything was normal. He then injected the mice with the drug *streptozotocin*, which destroyed the insulin-producing *beta islet* cells in the pancreas, thus inducing diabetes. Three weeks later, he once again dipped their feet in ink and had them walk across the paper. This time there was a noticeable difference in gait. Each rat's gait was no longer steady and firm, but showed wobbling and uneven contact with the paper, obvious symptoms of diabetic neuropathy. With time, the rats' toes spread apart without the power to pull them in and the arch of the foot disappeared, making the footprint on the white paper longer. The nerves were not functioning as they should.

Next, he took a second batch of normal rats and conducted nerve decompression surgery in which he removed the soft tissue surrounding the tarsal tunnel. He then replicated the technique of making them diabetic, dipped their feet in ink, and had this group walk across white paper. He repeated the ink/paper test every month for one year, which is half of the rat's lifetime. Lo and behold—the second group did not exhibit an unsteady gait. They'd regained their balance and sure-footedness. Even with blood sugars of 400 (normal being 90), the rats walked normally and did not develop diabetic walking patterns. From this Dellon concluded that nerve compression in the foot was the same as nerve compression in the wrist. It was diabetes-related damage to the rats' nerves that resulted in the swelling, constriction, and reduced blood flow seen in the first group.

He realized that "because it wasn't done" hadn't been a good enough reason. The very same procedure that was helping tens of thousands of people with their carpal tunnel pain could be used to relieve nerve compression in the tarsal tunnel and thus help diabetes patients with foot neuropathy. It was so simple a conclusion as to be profound.

His patient had been right to push—the nerves in the lower extremity were no different in that they too were being compressed and this compression was causing the pain and numbness. Rather than waiting for the compressed nerves to lead to gangrene and amputation, Dellon's decompression surgery could eliminate pain, restore blood flow to the nerves, and save his patient's foot.*

After speaking with Dr. Dellon and reading more about his procedure and his remarkable results, I traveled to Baltimore to learn how to perform surgical nerve decompression (neurolysis) of the tarsal (ankle) tunnel—formally known as the Dellon Triple Nerve Decompression. I'm proud and grateful that I was able to learn from the inventor himself.

My first nerve decompression surgery was on a patient named Diane, and we had amazing results. She'd been in extreme pain and was having tremendous difficulty walking and maintaining her balance. Peripheral neuropathy was severely limiting her quality of life. Had it progressed, she'd likely need an amputation. With the decompression surgery, she was soon up and walking. Her improvement was so astonishing that I knew this surgery could have a real impact on many of my patients.

A few months later, Diane was back in my office, this time with a cast on her arm. "What happened?" I asked.

"Well, it felt so good to be up and walking again, that I started exercising and feeling better. My husband and I decided to take a trip to Hawaii, and while we were out hiking, I slipped on a wet rock and broke my arm," she said with a smile.

---

*Dr. Dellon's first clinical paper on this concept was published in 1992.

She'd gone from being incapacitated in a wheelchair to hiking in Hawaii, which was very good news, even if it meant she'd slipped and broken her arm. Best of all, she had her quality of life back.

Since that time, I've performed more than 1,500 Dellon procedures, and none of my patients has had a serious complication from the surgery. By decompressing the nerves in the tarsal tunnel, we restore blood flow and nerve function to the foot. This is enough to help patients avoid the unnoticed damage to their feet that can lead to an infected ulcer. It's also enough to restore better blood flow and nerve function to the feet in general, so that they are less likely to be damaged in the first place. As a result, only two of these patients has ever had another ulceration in the treated foot and no one has gone on to have an amputation.

From Decompression Surgery to the Sugar Saga

So, while my success rate on ankles was similar to Dr. Dellon's, I wondered why we weren't able to reach 100 percent. And Dellon challenged me to figure it out. Reading the journal *Circulation*, I came across a 2004 article, "Asymmetrical Dimethylarginine: The Uber Marker?" by John Cooke, M.D., Ph.D. In this article, he examined the "burgeoning body of literature" that supported asymmetrical dimethylarginine (ADMA) as a master blood marker for endothelial vasodilator dysfunction,* a major contributor to coronary artery disease.

---

*An imbalance between the vasoconstricting (narrowing) and vasodilating (widening) substances within the inner lining (endothelium) of your blood vessels. Essentially, what controls your blood pressure when your heart beats.

Cooke was looking at risk factors for endovascular disease and noted that all of the traditional risk factors—diabetes, smoking, high blood pressure, and high cholesterol—are linked to constricted blood vessels. He noted that people with these higher risk factors also have more ADMA in their blood.

What makes this ADMA molecule so interesting? Well, I mentioned it earlier, in Chapter 2 when I discussed the nitric oxide pathway. While some ADMA is naturally produced, too much ADMA impacts the body's ability to convert L-arginine to nitric oxide. The result is constriction within the vessel, which dramatically reduces blood flow.

The Important Missing Link to Sugar

It was all beginning to fall into place. Key to the successful conversion of L-arginine to nitric oxide is something called the *tetrahydrobiopterin cofactor* (BH[4]), which is essential for various enzyme activities involving the vitamins C, B_6, B_{12}, and folic acid. BH(4) is a self-protecting factor for the nitric oxide pathway discussed in the previous chapter and it also provides a neurotransmitter-releasing function. This is significant because the chemistry of vitamin C and glucose are nearly identical—they're just two carbons off from one another. Insulin mediates both. The role of diabetes in the inflammation of the nerves I was surgically decompressing in the foot and ankle was beginning to come into view.

In the 1970s, Linus Pauling famously linked low vitamin C levels with cancer and heart disease. At about the same time, Dr. John Ely developed the glucose-ascorbate antagonism theory. This theory stated that glucose and vitamin

C compete against one another for the insulin they need to migrate into your cells and do their jobs.

In that competition, glucose trumps vitamin C. This means that the more glucose circulating in the blood, the less vitamin C will enter the cells. When vitamin C is missing from the B4 cofactor, your body will not convert L-arginine to nitric oxide. Instead, it will convert to peroxynitrite, causing excessive constriction of the endothelium and reduction in blood flow.

So what does that all mean in simple terms? Let's take the ever-present glass of orange juice on nearly everyone's breakfast table. When Pauling made his discovery linking low vitamin C levels with cancer, the orange juice producers successfully sold us on a big glass of orange juice as the healthy way to start the day. In reality, all that sugar in the orange juice can cancel out any benefit from the vitamin C. When you reach for that morning OJ, you've been taught to believe you're getting your essential vitamin C, but what you're really getting is—you guessed it, sugar.*

The Small Fiber/Large Fiber Neuropathy Disconnect

Decompression surgery has not been accepted by all physicians. Primarily this is because of the widespread and misguided belief that small fiber and large fiber neuropathy are not related. The reason for this misconception dates back to the 1800s, when neuropathies were being discovered. The

---

*An 8-ounce glass of orange juice can contain as much as 21 grams of sugar, while a whole orange contains 9 grams plus 2.3 grams of fiber. And fiber is the bonus prize.

naming process for the newly defined conditions had the same flaw we see throughout medicine. The names described *effects* only and the names stuck: Morton's neuroma, Bell's palsy, and many others. However, all the body's nerves are connected and inflammation leading to compression is the underlying cause of many seemingly unrelated illnesses. Remember, physicians generally learn in silos related to their disciplines and it's human nature to trust what you were taught by those early professors you respected. It's human nature to be rigid in your long-held beliefs; it's scientific to challenge them.

Let's Connect the Dots

As we've discussed, most people with elevated sugars will develop neuropathy. The first nerves to be affected are the *small fiber nerves*, also known as C fiber nerves. Small fiber nerves don't have a myelin sheath—the fatty layer that wraps around larger nerves and has very much the same function as insulation on an electrical wire. Small fiber nerves are unmyelinated, mostly because they don't need a lot of energy to do their work. The small fiber nerves are found in the skin and organs. They mostly control autonomic visceral functions: heart rate, digestion, respiratory system, and the function of other internal organs, such as your bladder. In your feet, they control sensation in the skin.

The next nerve fibers to be affected by peripheral neuropathy are the *sensory fibers*. These are the nerves that communicate pain or a change in sensation of a body part (toe, finger, whatever). Because transmitting these signals requires more energy, these nerves need insulation, so they're myelinated.

The latter phases of neuropathy affect motor function—

the nerves that move your muscles and joints. These are *large fibers* that conduct the most energy and require the thickest myelin.

To understand this distinction let's talk about how we measure things that are very small. The unit of measurement is called the *micron*, represented by the Greek letter μ. A red blood cell is 8μ in diameter. Pure small fiber neuropathy is a rare condition in which only the tiniest nerve fibers, those without myelin (0.5 to 1.5μ in diameter), and thinly myelinated nerve fibers (1 to 2μ in diameter) that transmit the perception of burning pain and heat (unmyelinated) and pricking pain and cold (thinly myelinated), are affected. In small fiber neuropathy you would have burning, stabbing pain and you'd feel as if your foot were on fire. You wouldn't have the numbness, buzzing, and tingling related to the larger myelinated fibers (5 to 15μ in diameter).

However, most of my patients have not only burning pain and numbness but tingling as well. This means they have both large and small fiber neuropathy, a multiple neuropathy—not a small fiber neuropathy. Indeed, in 1986 Dellon and colleagues actually proved that chronic nerve compression in humans causes a *mixed mono-neuropathy*—with chronic nerve compression, in which both the small and large myelinated fibers are affected.

I had a patient who came to me after he'd been traveling in Israel. While there, he'd gone with a friend for a barefoot walk on the beach. The friend couldn't walk without sandals, complaining the sand was too hot, while my patient shrugged it off.

"Don't be so whiny; this isn't hot."

The sand was hot; he just couldn't feel it. And he got some pretty ugly blisters. When he returned home, he got a full workup to find out what was wrong, but his doctors couldn't find anything. I did a skin biopsy and discovered that he was losing cells in the nerves in his feet. He was experiencing symptoms of small fiber neuropathy. Mind you, this was not a diagnosis; it was still just a description. We hadn't discovered *what* was causing the trouble.

The next time he returned he was limping. He told me that the pain and the limp "comes and goes." Within a month he couldn't walk. This time we did a full MRI and, lo and behold, we discovered a thoracic tumor in his chest cavity. In medical language this is called a "space-occupying lesion." This lesion was causing a compression on his nerve, which resulted in the neuropathy in his feet.

I tell you this story because it shows that compressions of your nerves can quickly slide you from small fiber neuropathy to large fiber neuropathy. In general, they are not separate and distinct diseases. There are some very distinct small fiber genetic diseases, which are not part of this paradigm—and these are the zebras.

The principle is called Occam's razor—the simplest of all options is most often the truth. For example, if you hear hooves, you think of horses—not zebras. In most cases small fiber and large fiber neuropathy are on a continuum, not separate and distinct pathologies. That means you should be looking for what connects them; you should be looking for horses. The genetic anomaly is the zebra. And we in the medical field should not be basing our assumptions on zebras when ninety-nine times out of a hundred we will be dealing with horses.

Global Compression Once More

All of this brings me back to global compression. We have much evidence that carbohydrates (including all sugars, as well as "starches" and alcohol that convert to sugar) cause inflammation. This and what to do about it will be the subject of future chapters.

In nerves, sugar-induced inflammation creeps slowly to compression and fibrosis. That trauma (or trauma experienced in other ways, such as contact sports) leads to pain and dysfunction, and since nerves are nerves, whether small fiber or large fiber, the pain and dysfunction can manifest anywhere in your body. In Chapter 4 we'll explore diseases you may never have considered as being influenced by diet.

4

Slightly Diabetic

THE METABOLIC SYNDROME
AND ITS UGLY COUSINS

Several years ago, a young woman came to see me because she was experiencing symptoms of phase 1 neuropathy: tingling, pain, and intermittent numbness in her feet.

Maria was obese, but her blood sugar wasn't elevated. When I asked about her diet and specifically if she ate sugar, she told me that everyone in her family got diabetes, usually by their forties.

"I eat all the sugar I can, while I still can," she joked.

I was taken aback. When I asked her to explain what she meant, she said that her doctor had told her diabetes was genetic and she couldn't avoid it. With that thinking in mind, she'd decided to eat all the sugar she could because she'd have to stop when she finally got sick. This was wrongheaded and dangerous. In her mind, she was *stocking up* on her pleasures. In reality, she was creating a sugar-laden environment that was pushing her ever more rapidly down the road to a disease she could easily avoid.

She was a real estate agent and in the middle of her busy season—and she'd only come to me because the pain was interfering with her work. Aside from her feet, she felt fine. I explained the path to diabetes and heart disease, gave her advice on foot care and pain management with over-the-counter analgesics, and asked her to see me again in three months. She made the return appointment on her way out, but she didn't keep it.

When my office manager followed up a few weeks later, we learned Maria had died from sudden cardiac arrest. She didn't believe her early-phase neuropathy needed to be taken seriously or that diabetes and heart disease were lurking just around the corner. Death is a horrible symptom.

Prediabetes

In the previous chapter I mentioned that type 2 diabetes is a conformational disease, meaning that by the time you may be diagnosed, the damage has already begun. And because of this long-term progression, observant doctors noticed that some patients have a constellation of health problems that, when combined, almost invariably lead to both type 2 diabetes and heart disease. In medicine, a group of signs and symptoms that frequently appear together is called a *syndrome* and so in 1988, the noted diabetes physician and researcher Gerald Reaven finally gave it a name: *syndrome X*. Today it's generally called the *metabolic syndrome*, because all the risk factors affect metabolism (the chemical processes that occur within your body to keep you alive). To make things even more confusing, metabolic syndrome is also associated with or even referred to as *prediabetes* or *insulin resistance*. Whatever the name, the syndrome is represented by glucose levels higher than normal, but below clinical diabetes.

Markers for the metabolic syndrome include:

- Obesity.
- Family history of diabetes.
- High triglycerides. These tiny fat droplets play a large role in putting on weight, clogging your arteries, increasing inflammation, and, as you will learn in subsequent chapters, directly causing neuropathy.
- High blood pressure (hypertension) or taking medication to treat it. If your blood pressure is 130/85 or higher or if you're already taking medication to lower it, you're showing one of the classic symptoms of the metabolic syndrome.
- Low HDL cholesterol. HDL is the so-called good cholesterol, because it helps remove the "bad" LDL cholesterol from your blood. Having HDL cholesterol less than 50 mg/dL* for a woman, or less than 40 mg/dL for a man, is a sign of the metabolic syndrome.
- High fasting blood sugar or taking medication to treat high blood sugar. This is the most significant sign of the metabolic syndrome. If your fasting blood sugar is consistently high, or if you're already taking medication to bring it down, you have the metabolic syndrome.
- The American Diabetes Association cites the following fasting blood sugar levels:
  - normal—at less than 100 mg/dL and preferably between 75 and 80 mg/dL
  - prediabetes—at 100-125 mg/dL
  - diabetes—at 126 mg/dL or higher.

---

*mg/dL is the unit of measurement for mass concentration of a substance in a liquid or gas (in this case blood). It stands for *milligrams per deciliter*. One tablespoon is approximately 15 milligrams. Approximately 6.76 tablespoons equals one deciliter.

If you have two of the five markers for the metabolic syndrome, you're now in the same dangerous health situation as about 25 percent of all American adults—and 40 percent of American adults over age fifty. You're well on your way to becoming one of the 26 million people who have type 2 diabetes. Down the road you can look forward to neuropathy, eye problems, kidney disease, and premature death from heart disease.*

We have decades of research indicating that, for the most part, obesity, lifestyle, diet, and stress contribute significantly to the progression of metabolic syndrome to the onset of type 2—and the eventual demise of a perfectly functioning pancreas. If we were in a poker game, it would be as if someone with type 1 diabetes had been dealt a poor genetic hand and played it brilliantly, while someone with type 2 had been dealt a brilliant genetic hand and played it poorly.

Riding the Blood Sugar Roller Coaster

When you eat a diet heavy in processed foods full of wheat and refined sugar, your body is put on a glucose roller coaster. Because fiber has been stripped out of these products, the sugar inherent in all carbohydrates literally enters the bloodstream in a rush. As your blood sugar spikes, most of the excess gets carried away to be stored as abdominal fat. While that's happening, excess glucose still circulates throughout your body, attaching itself to proteins (glycating) and building up sorbitol in the cells, causing them to swell and

---

*Sixty-five percent of patients having a first heart attack also have the metabolic syndrome.

compress the nerves.* So even without a formal diagnosis of diabetes, presence of the metabolic syndrome means that your nerves are becoming inflamed, building up scar tissue, and compressing. This process can manifest first in diseases other than diabetes. In earlier chapters I mentioned carpal tunnel syndrome, migraines, and other illnesses for which science is building a strong body of evidence connecting them to nerve compression.

As I apply the relationship of sugar and global compression theory to my patients, an ever-increasing number of diseases come into view. After all, nerves are nerves regardless of where they are in the body. Studies on some of these relationships are just beginning. For example, the ninth cranial (glossopharyngeal) nerve is implicated in the relatively rare and catastrophic amyotrophic lateral sclerosis (ALS). From my viewpoint, ALS is a compression neuropathy, and interestingly, there is growing attention to neurodegenerative diseases (such as ALS) found in professional football players.† Researchers with the U.S. Centers for Disease Control and Prevention and the National Institute for Occupational Safety and Health reported that the incidence of ALS was four times higher in National Football League players than in the general population. In response to this and other studies, the NFL announced a $30 million donation to the National Institutes of Health for research into the increased risk of neurodegenerative disease among football players.

---

*As mentioned in Chapter 3, early observations that patients with diabetes were susceptible to chronic compression of the peripheral nerves were what first piqued Dellon's interest and led him to the conclusion that "decompressing" this nerve would relieve the pain.

†Similar research has been conducted among boxers and soccer players.

What does this have to do with sugar? A great deal when you recognize that professional athletes consume a tremendous number of carbohydrates* besides experiencing repetitive microtrauma to the cranial nerves.

And Now, the Ugly Cousins

The following are diseases you may not associate with diet or sugar; however, I believe the evidence is mounting that these have origins in keeping with the global compression theory.

$$
\begin{array}{ccc}
\text{(Carbohydrates)} & & \textbf{Chronic} \\
\text{Sugar} \quad = & \textbf{Inflammation} & + \quad \text{Trauma} \\
& & \textbf{(Compression} \\
& & \textbf{or Injury)}
\end{array}
$$

$$
= \quad \text{Nerve Damage, Pain, and Dysfunction}
$$
$$
\textbf{(of Any Peripheral Nerve)}
$$

Alzheimer's Disease

Despite much research, this devastating illness still is poorly understood and essentially untreatable. In fact, it can't be diagnosed accurately while the patient is alive. Only an autopsy can find the tangled proteins in the brain that are characteristic of the disease.

Early in the disease, and before other major symptoms have developed, people with Alzheimer's often lose their

---

*How much carbohydrate is up for debate, but a study in *Sports Medicine* cited a range of 5–7 grams of carbohydrate (CHO) per kilogram of body weight per day to 7–10 g/kg/day for endurance athletes. For a 300-pound NFL lineman, that could mean 682–1,364 grams of CHO depending upon whether or not it was game day. That's a lot of carbs.

sense of smell. Doctors sometimes use the peanut butter test to help in their diagnoses. If the patient can't detect the odor of peanut butter when it's held right under his or her nose, Alzheimer's is a likely cause. Is the loss of smell related to compression of the olfactory nerve? I believe it is.

This nerve, also known as the *first cranial* nerve, reaches the nose through a very tight tunnel that runs along the *ethmoid* bone, the bone in the skull that separates the nasal cavity from the brain. The nerve passes through many tiny openings in the *cribriform* plate of the bone, a structure that forms the roof of the nasal cavity and looks a bit like a sieve. The *hippocampus*, the brain's memory center, is also part of the olfactory nerve nucleus. Those centers are intermingled, so the two symptoms are intertwined. First you lose your sense of smell and then you lose your memory.

I often think back to an anesthesiologist I worked with on many surgeries. He was in his fifties, overweight, and had type 2 diabetes. Surgery on television is very tidy—the blood is hardly ever shown, and of course the smells of the operating room are missing. In reality, surgery involves a lot of blood and a lot of *electrocautery*—burning—to stop it. The smell of burned flesh is distinctive. Even more distinctive is the horrible smell of rotting meat that comes from a gangrenous foot. Lots of anesthesiologists try to avoid these cases, but the one I'm thinking of never did. He claimed not to notice the smell of rotted flesh. His lack of a strong sense of smell in his early fifties was, to me, a clue that he was already suffering from the earliest signs of Alzheimer's disease, even if he didn't know it and had no other symptoms. I wasn't surprised to learn that he ended up retiring early and died in his late sixties from complications of the disease.

Alzheimer's, Diabetes, and Global Compression

The loss of smell as a harbinger to Alzheimer's is another example of how global compression from sugar is actually the underlying cause of very different symptoms. Sugar contributes to compression of the olfactory nerve just as it contributes to compression elsewhere. And we know that people with type 2 diabetes are at least twice as likely to develop dementia or Alzheimer's disease as are people without diabetes. Some researchers, such as the neuropathologist Suzanne de la Monte of Alpert Medical School, Brown University, believe that Alzheimer's is actually a form of diabetes—which they call type 3. When brain cells become resistant to insulin, the neurons don't get enough fuel and deteriorate, causing memory loss, confusion, and other typical symptoms of dementia. In addition, the high glucose levels that result may be the cause of the characteristic protein plaques that damage the brain in Alzheimer's disease.

There's no cure for Alzheimer's disease and no drug that does anything useful to treat the symptoms. We can't even say for sure how to avoid the disease, because your risk increases with aging. It stands to reason, however, that there's a simple way to limit your risk of getting any chronic disease that might be related to sugar consumption: stop eating it.

Morton's Neuroma

Morton's neuroma is a fairly common foot problem. A patient will often tell me it feels like she has a pebble stuck in the ball of her foot, between the third and fourth toes. She may also experience severe sharp or burning pain in the ball of the foot; the toes may be painful or numb.

When Dr. Thomas George Morton of the Pennsylvania Hospital in Philadelphia (where I trained) first described the condition way back in 1876, he thought it might be due to a damaged metatarsal joint in the toe, because his first patient injured the foot hiking. His name for this was "metatarsalgia." He amputated the toe. The pathologist found no problem with the joint. The patient got better and Morton realized it was because he had also removed the nerves to the digit.

The neuroma part of the name got attached to the condition later when researchers thought that the thickening sometimes seen in the affected nerve was a type of benign tumor. In 1992, Dellon described this swelling on the nerve as being related to chronic compression and that the best form of treatment was not excision of a "neuroma" but rather a *neurolysis*, or release of pressure on the compressed *interdigital nerve*.

Most so-called Morton's neuromas of the foot are caused by mechanical pressure. However, in a study involving my Morton's neuroma patients, I found that 42 percent had either the metabolic syndrome or diabetes.

Plantar Fasciitis

Besides Morton's neuroma, *plantar fasciitis* is another common foot condition—this time an inflammation of the *plantar fascia*, the thick band of fibrous tissue that runs along the bottom of your foot and connects your heel bone (the *calcaneus*) to your toes. Plantar fasciitis can cause intense, stabbing heel pain.

Marathon runners and other heavy-duty athletes often get plantar fasciitis from all the stress they put on their feet.

Most of my patients, however, are overweight and in their fifties or older. Few ever ran a marathon; none do so now. Importantly, many also have gait abnormalities that put extra stress on the plantar fascia. And when I ask them about blood sugar, they almost always tell me it's high. When I check the feet of a plantar fasciitis patient for peripheral neuropathy, I often find that she's in the early phases.

Are you starting to see the pattern here? Plantar fasciitis is a compression neuropathy—a compression of the *lateral plantar* nerve in the tarsal tunnel. The fascia doesn't conduct nerve impulses and it's not the source of the pain. What makes the foot hurt in plantar fasciitis is the fascia pressing on swollen nerves. Yet another way your body can tell you that you're eating too much sugar.

Not every doctor agrees with me when I contend that both plantar fasciitis and Morton's neuroma are directly related to excess sugar. In fact, most will disagree. And yet few have had my experience in successfully treating these conditions with dietary changes. Is that controversial? You bet it is. Today it's rare when I perform the standard surgical treatment for Morton's neuroma—and I don't hesitate telling colleagues they're wrong to continue doing it. On the other hand, I've had grateful calls from primary care physicians because I was able to help their patients crippled by foot pain get better without surgery—and improve their diabetes at the same time. The bottom line? My job is to help my patients. If that's controversial, so be it.

Success with conditions I see most often led me to wonder if other chronic diseases like multiple sclerosis (MS) would improve if sugar and carbohydrates were sharply reduced or eliminated from the diet.

Multiple Sclerosis

MS is a devastating, chronic neurological disease that affects the central nervous system—the brain and spinal cord. In MS, the myelin sheath, which wraps around the nerve fibers, is gradually destroyed in multiple places by lesions that damage the myelin and leave scars behind. Just as a break in the insulation around an electrical wire causes short circuits, damage to the myelin sheath of a nerve causes muscle weakness, contractions, and pain, among other symptoms.

First described by the great French neurologist Jean-Martin Charcot in 1868, multiple sclerosis is usually classified as an autoimmune disease; but there's no known cause, and no known cure. Treatment of MS focuses on managing the symptoms, but the many different drugs used usually aren't all that effective, nor do they help for long. Others may work well but can cause dangerous side effects. Tysabri (natalizumab), for instance, is a monoclonal antibody that can help cut back on exacerbations (periods when the disease is worse) and slow progression; but this comes at the risk of progressive multifocal leukoencephalopathy (PML), a viral infection of the brain that usually leads to death or severe disability. If a drug like that is being seriously considered for your treatment, isn't it time to look into other possibilities?

A few years ago, I attended a conference on MS, and there I was introduced to a theory developed by Paolo Zamboni, a professor of medicine at the University of Ferrara in Italy. His wife had been diagnosed with MS in 1995 and he'd spent many years looking for a way to help her. Then, in 2008, he hypothesized that MS is not an autoimmune disease, as is widely believed, but rather is a vascular disease. Zamboni believed that a compromised flow of blood in the veins draining the central nervous system plays a role in the development of the disease. He termed this phenomenon *chronic cerebrospinal venous insufficiency* (CCSVI) and devised a procedure using a small balloon (angioplasty) to widen the passage in the jugular vein. To his utter joy, the procedure alleviated his wife's symptoms. That made me think about what might be happening. The *vagus nerve* lies right on top of the *jugular vein*. When Zamboni widened (dilated) the vein, the symptoms subsided.

The procedure is not without its critics, as reported by Paul Tullis in his *New York Times* article, "A Controversial Cure for M.S." These include Florian Doepp, a neurologist at Charité Hospital in Berlin, who finds "no evidence to support" CCSVI in MS or the surgical treatment of such. And yet when I look at the CCSVI procedure through the lens of compression, I think it makes sense.

My own hypothesis is that the ADMA (discussed in Chapter 2), which makes the endothelium sticky, is causing compromised blood flow to the brain, or that perhaps the vagus nerve, because of the ADMA, is stuck to the jugular vein. Then, when you inflate the vein and expand the tunnel, it could unstick the vagus nerve, stopping the symptoms. The recurrence rate is fairly high with the Zamboni procedure, which could actually reinforce the idea that a diet high in sugar and the resulting sticky ADMA is the real problem.

Several other scientists continue to research CCSVI and venous angioplasty, including neurologist David Hubbard and his wife, Arlene. After learning their son had MS, the Hubbards established a foundation to support research into ways to improve venous drainage and avoiding foods causing inflammation.

In most cases, MS symptoms come and go in a phase of the disease called relapsing-remitting. The symptoms gradually get worse, however, and many people with MS end up disabled and in wheelchairs. That's what happened to Terry Wahls, M.D., a specialist in internal medicine and professor at the University of Iowa Carver College of Medicine, who was diagnosed with MS in 2000. Using her skills as a talented physician and researcher, she pored over all the studies of treatment for chronic brain diseases and quickly came to the conclusion that some nutrients are particularly important for brain health. So she began taking them as supplements. The supplements slowed her disease but didn't stop it. The next step was to replace the nutritional supplements with the whole foods that contain the nutrients. Not surprisingly, this turned out to be the answer. In December 2007, Dr. Wahls began an experiment on herself, which she later named the Wahls Protocol. Within a year, she was out of her wheelchair, walking without a cane, and back to riding her bike and practicing medicine.

The Link with Autism

In the year 2000, approximately 16 people per 10,000 were diagnosed with autism. Today, the ratio is closer to one in 50. There is obviously a tremendous environmental impact that has affected the numbers so dramatically in that short time frame.

Delayed speech is one of the most significant symptoms of autism. The nerve that operates speech is the *hypoglossal nerve*, otherwise known as *cranial nerve number 12*. Studies have found that the brain stem tunnel on autistic children is 1.1 millimeters more narrow than a normal brain stem tunnel. Because scientists know when an embryo's organs develop at each stage of a pregnancy, they can pinpoint exactly when a malformation occurs. On day 22 of gestation (often before a woman even knows she's pregnant) the HoxA1 gene puts down two proteins as the hypoglossal nerve is developed and the nervous system is starting to form. That's all this gene does and it does it only on this one specific day. If the gene fails to put down those two proteins on that day, the result is this 1.1-millimeter-smaller brain stem tunnel. If the hypoglossal nerve is compressed within a smaller tunnel, then the muscle that it supplies with nerves—in this case, the tongue—does not function properly, and the result can be a delay in speech.

We don't know exactly what causes this to happen, but based on research by Dr. Stephanie Seneff, a senior research scientist at the Massachusetts Institute of Technology, on the impact of genetically modified organisms on the *shikimate pathway* (a crucial metabolic pathway in bacteria), I suspect that we are eating something that is changing the bacteria in our guts. This causes "leaky gut" syndrome, a condition where the walls of the intestines become more permeable than they should be. Undigested food particles and bacteria can slip through and enter the bloodstream, causing a range of health problems. I suspect that if the mother has a leaky gut, the HoxA1 gene is somehow being prevented from doing its job and the fetus is affected.

Sugar and Cancer

I treat many patients who are both over sixty and have long-standing type 2 diabetes. Over the years, many of these patients have also developed cancer. That's not a coincidence or because my patients tend to be older. It's because people with diabetes are much more likely to get cancer—something that's been tracked by the American Institute for Cancer Research for decades. If you have diabetes, your risk of cancer of the liver, pancreas, and endometrium (in women) is at least twice as high as for someone who is like you but without type 2 diabetes. Your risk of colon cancer, breast cancer, and bladder cancer is about 1.2 to 1.5 times higher. The only cancer that has a slightly lower risk for people with diabetes is prostate cancer.

Not only are you more likely to get cancer if you have type 2 diabetes, but you're much more likely to die of it. Women with both breast cancer and diabetes are about 35 percent more likely to die of the cancer than are women without diabetes. Overall, women with diabetes have an 11 percent greater chance of dying from cancer; men with diabetes have a 17 percent greater risk.

Like normal cells, cancer cells have receptors for insulin and something called *insulin-like growth factor* (IGF-1). Because cancer cells grow rapidly in an uncontrolled manner, they need a lot of glucose to fuel such expansion. When your blood sugar is high and you've got a lot of insulin sloshing around, you're giving the cancer cells exactly what they need to grow and spread.*

The incidence of cancer in the United States and around the world has been increasing at a staggering rate. This increase tracks right along with the increase in refined sugars, carbohydrates, and high-fructose corn syrup in the diet—which, in turn, correlates with the explosive growth of

---

*In addition, IGF-1 itself also seems to stimulate the growth of cancer cells.

obesity (an independent risk factor for cancer) and type 2 diabetes. It's not a coincidence—the massive increase in our intake of sugar, especially HFCS, is tied to our increasing levels of cancer.

Think of it this way. When a cancer patient gets a PET scan after treatment, the physician is looking for energy hot spots, places where there is more sugar in the cell. More sugar means there is more cancer eating it. It's like a kitchen with a pile of sugar on the floor. You flip on the light and see roaches, so you spray the heck out of them with insecticide and kill them (chemotherapy). But if you don't get rid of the sugar, what happens next? The roaches come back.

PART II

The Train to Nowhere

5

On Track for Nerve Damage

ARE YOUR NERVES ALREADY INFLAMED?

In the Why Should I Read This Book? Quiz, I asked you to identify a few simple conditions that could indicate you're already experiencing the negative effects of sugar in your diet. Now I want to explore those precursors in depth.

The thirteen simple questions below will help you determine if you're already on the way to nerve damage and type 2 diabetes, and the debilitating neuropathy that comes with it. I call it the "itis" and "ectomy" quiz because so many of the medical diagnoses you've already received are actually the result of nerve inflammation precipitated by excess sugar intake. You'll recognize a couple of the topics from earlier chapters.

The "Itis" and "Ectomy" Quiz

1. Is your waist larger than 35 inches if you're a woman or 40 inches if you're a man?
    ☐ Yes   ☐ No

2. Do you get frequent headaches (more than two a week) or migraines or did you experience migraines in your teens or twenties?

☐ Yes   ☐ No

3. Do you wake up with tingling (often with itching and burning) or numbness in the fingers of one or both hands—or have you ever been diagnosed with carpal tunnel syndrome?

☐ Yes   ☐ No

4. Do you often have a runny nose, sinus headaches, or need to take over-the-counter or prescription antihistamines (drugs such as Allegra and Claritin)? Have you been diagnosed with chronic sinusitis?

☐ Yes   ☐ No

5. Do you feel tired most or all of the time?

☐ Yes   ☐ No

6. Did you have severe acne as a teenager or do you have adult acne (more than the occasional blemish) now?

☐ Yes   ☐ No

7. Do your feet sometimes feel itchy, burning, tingling, or numb?

☐ Yes   ☐ No

8. Have you ever had gingivitis, periodontal disease, or a root canal?

☐ Yes   ☐ No

9. Do you have skin tags or dark, velvety areas on your skin?

☐ Yes   ☐ No

10. Are your legs sometimes restless at night (a crawling or creeping sensation relieved by moving)?

☐ Yes   ☐ No

11. Have you ever had a gallbladder attack or had your gall-bladder removed?

☐ Yes   ☐ No

12. Do you have frequent (more than two times a week) heartburn, upset stomach, constipation, or diarrhea?

☐ Yes   ☐ No

13. Do you get frequent (more than once a year) bladder or yeast infections?

☐ Yes   ☐ No

SCORING

Your score indicates risk and how quickly you are moving toward disease and debility.

1 to 3 Yes answers: Your risk is real but low.

4 to 6 Yes answers: Your risk is moderate, but immediate action to change your diet can reduce it.

More than 6 Yes answers: You may already have prediabetes or diabetes and could be far down the path to severe neuropathy. See your doctor as soon as possible.

What Your Answers Mean

Now that you've completed the "Itis" and "Ectomy" Quiz, you may be wondering why I'm so interested in your waist size, your headaches, and your skin—let alone your gallbladder. While the various health issues in the quiz seem to be different, they're actually all connected by one common denominator: sugar consumption. Every one of the quiz questions is designed to explore end organs most easily impacted by high sugar consumption—and to determine how far along you are toward killing your nerves.

1. Is your waist larger than 35 inches if you're a woman or 40 inches if you're a man?

A large waist indicates you're significantly overweight and probably have become resistant to the effects of insulin. This means your blood sugar is almost certainly higher than it should be—and, in turn, means damage to your nerves has already begun.

The risk factors for metabolic syndrome were discussed in Chapter 4 and you officially have the syndrome if you have at least two out of five risk factors: obesity, high triglycerides, high blood pressure, low HDL cholesterol, and a high fasting blood sugar (glucose) count. Of these, obesity (as represented by a large waist size) is usually the first factor to present itself.

Did you just wake up with this condition one morning? No. Obesity creeps up on you through years of a diet high in sugar and refined carbohydrates, combined with a sedentary lifestyle. If you're still in the early stages of the metabolic syndrome, it's possible to retrace your steps and get on a healthier path.

Step one?

Delete the sugar from your diet.

2. Do you get frequent headaches (more than two a week) or migraines or did you experience migraines in your teens or twenties?

If you get frequent headaches, there's too much sugar in your diet—and your body isn't handling it very well. As discussed in the last chapter, when glucose floods your bloodstream, this triggers a surge of insulin to clear it away. And in the early stages of the process, your body can respond by overshooting the mark, thus removing too much glucose from your blood. You may then become hypoglycemic—your blood sugar drops below normal. (This can also sometimes happen if you skip a meal.) The most common symptoms of hypoglycemia are headaches and cravings for sugary or starchy foods. You might then eat a second candy bar, which will raise your blood sugar back up to normal and relieve the headache—all at the cost of starting the whole cycle again.

Just as a quick drop in blood sugar is a common trigger for headache, it's also a trigger for a migraine, but for a somewhat different reason.

Migraines

A migraine is a severe, often incapacitating headache frequently accompanied by nausea and sensitivity to light—it's a headache with a vengeance. Migraines can be caused by many things, including hormonal changes, stress, low blood sugar from missed meals, and food allergies. The occasional migraine headache is manageable, but some people are chronic sufferers—and migraines experienced more than once a month can seriously disrupt their lives. Women are three times more likely to experience a migraine than are men. In fact, about 20 percent of all women have experienced at least one migraine headache (often in adolescence).* In all, 36 million Americans, or 12 percent of the population, get migraines at least once a year.

---

*The exception is the rare and more severe *cluster migraine*, which is six times more likely to occur in men.

Drugs for frequent migraines have the same problem as drugs for peripheral neuropathy—they don't work very well and have serious side effects. And yet, for some people with chronic migraines, surgical decompression of select nerves in the face or scalp can reduce the frequency of the headaches or even eliminate them. The observation leading to this concept was first made by Dr. Bahman Guyuron, a plastic surgeon in Cleveland. After brow lift surgery, a patient told him she no longer got migraines. Because this procedure involves releasing the *supraorbital nerve* (one of several cranial nerves associated with frequent migraines), Guyuron began offering the surgery to migraine sufferers—with outstanding results. Since then, research has confirmed that decompressing other nerves causing migraines (such as the *occipital nerves* that control the top and back of the scalp) can provide almost instant relief.

And for the Truly "Bad Seed"

If chronic migraine headaches are bad, *trigeminal neuralgia* is much worse. The *trigeminal nerve* (also known as the fifth cranial nerve) has three main branches that control sensation in the face. Sometimes one or more branches get compressed and become agonizingly painful and disabling. Before the development of effective treatment, trigeminal neuralgia was even labeled "the suicide disease" because of the numbers of people taking their own lives rather than enduring the pain. It usually surfaces after the age of forty and affects women in a ratio of 2:1. The nerve compression seems to come from an enlarged blood vessel pressing on the nerve (where it originates at the base of the brain), and as with other types of nerve compression, drugs don't help much. Some patients turn to microvascular decompression, a surgical procedure that involves opening the skull, looking for the spot where the blood vessel presses on the trigeminal nerve, and placing a tiny bit of soft material between the blood vessel and the nerve.

This extremely effective technique was pioneered by Dr. Peter Jannetta, and you won't be surprised to learn that for many years it was extremely controversial. Today Jannetta's approach is widely used to treat not only the devastating effects of trigeminal neuralgia, but also other conditions originating from compressed nerves.*

Needless to say, while the Jannetta procedure is safe and effective, brain surgery isn't to be taken lightly. Fortunately, for many patients there is now another option that doesn't involve opening up your skull and that has basically no risk of death, stroke, infection, or facial numbness. New developments in radiation treatment let doctors target very small, specific areas of the brain with a onetime blast of gamma rays, which shrink the nerve, relieve compression, and eliminate pain.

Sugar-Triggered Migraine

Step one in triggering a migraine with sugar is eating a lot of it. As with headaches, this can cause first a surge in insulin and then a drop in blood sugar. When blood sugar drops quickly, the arteries in the head may not get enough glucose to fuel them properly. In people prone to migraines, low blood sugar can make the arteries spasm and constrict. In addition, the body compensates for low blood sugar by constricting arteries to raise blood pressure. This reduces blood flow even more and contributes to the migraine.

---

*These include Ménière's disease (an inner ear disorder causing disabling vertigo) and tinnitus (ringing in the ears).

Recent research has shown that people who are prone to migraines also often have elevated levels of insulin in their blood.* This happens because they have become resistant to the effects of insulin, and so to *force* glucose into their cells, they need to produce extra insulin. This excess insulin can in turn cause a migraine because it interferes with the action of the nitric oxide pathway.†

If you get migraines, you may have noticed that you crave carbohydrates just before the attack begins. You may even have learned to short-circuit the migraine by eating something sweet or starchy when you first feel it coming on. You may also have recognized that you're more likely to get a migraine if you skip a meal, which can lead to a drop in your blood sugar. Two obvious approaches will help keep your blood sugar on an even keel: limit your intake of sugary or starchy food and eat regular, low-carb meals. It's not a guarantee, but usually, no trigger means no migraine.

The story of sugar and migraines actually begins with Thomas Willis, a seventeenth-century physician considered the father of modern neurology.‡ Willis had a patient and mistress named Lady Anne Conway, a renowned British philosopher who'd suffered from incapacitating migraines most of her life. She sought relief everywhere, even going so far as to have her jugular veins opened to relieve pressure. None of

---

*A condition known as *hyperinsulinemia*.

†Identified in Chapter 2 as one of the three key chemical pathways, nitric oxide is necessary to make your blood vessels relax so blood can flow smoothly through them. Block the pathway by having too much insulin in your bloodstream and the small arteries in the head can become constricted, leading to a migraine.

‡*Gray's Anatomy* still uses the term "circle of Willis" in describing the blood vessels in the brain.

the treatments she endured helped and she died at age forty-seven. Willis conducted an autopsy on Lady Conway and recorded that her brain tissue was "swollen and scarred."

Because Lady Conway was an aristocrat, her diet most certainly included the expensive treat of seventeenth-century London—sugar. Was this an early indication that inflammation and the resulting scarring could have played a part in her condition? Could the sugar in her diet have been a factor in her migraines? That's what I hypothesize—Willis to Jannetta to Dellon. All paths lead to global compression, inflammation of the nerves caused by sugar.

3. **Do you wake up with tingling (often with itching and burning) or numbness in the fingers of one or both hands—or have you ever been diagnosed with carpal tunnel syndrome?**

Tingling (often with itching and burning) and numbness in the fingers are classic symptoms of carpal tunnel syndrome (CTS), a painful condition caused by compression of the *median nerve*, one of the three main nerves that run down the arm and into the hand. The median nerve controls movement and sensation in your thumb and all the other fingers except half of the ring finger, and the pinkie, which are controlled by the ulnar nerve.

The median nerve passes into the hand through a narrow tunnel in your wrist. The floor of the tunnel is formed by the carpal (wrist) bones; the sides are formed by tendons; and the roof is formed by the transverse carpal ligament. Because the tunnel is narrow and formed by bones, tendons, and ligaments—the toughest tissues in your body—anything that makes the nerve swell up will also squeeze it, because the swollen nerve can't expand against the tougher tissue. The nerve gets compressed in place by its own swelling. Step on a hose and you slow or stop the flow of water; compress a nerve and you do much the same thing to the impulses that flow back and forth along it.

CTS is a form of *mononeuropathy*, or neuropathy that affects only a single nerve. Like all neuropathies, it usually starts gradually, with only occasional minor discomfort and then progresses to chronic itching, tingling, burning, and numbness. The symptoms gradually worsen, causing increasing discomfort and loss of strength in the hand. The condition is sometimes caused by an injury or repetitive motion, and sometimes simply by having a smaller carpal tunnel than usual. However, I believe that in most cases, compression of the median nerve is the direct result of the inflammation caused by sugar. And even distinguished public health sites such as that established by the University of Maryland Medical Center advise CTS patients to "avoid refined foods such as white bread, pasta, and sugar."

Carpal Tunnel and Diabetes

The link between CTS and diabetes was established as early as 1930 and continues to be explored by researchers such as Martin Gulliford of King's College London. So, when I ask if you're having any symptoms of carpal tunnel syndrome, or if you've already been diagnosed with it, I'm really asking if your diet is high in sugar. I'm also asking indirectly if you already have the metabolic syndrome, since carpal tunnel syndrome is more common among people who are obese.

Among metabolically normal people, the incidence of CTS is roughly 2 percent of the population. Among those already diagnosed with diabetes but with no signs yet of diabetic polyneuropathy, the incidence of CTS is 14 percent. And among people with diabetes *and* polyneuropathy, the incidence of CTS is a whopping 30 percent. The longer you have diabetes, the more likely you are to develop CTS. Sugar causes global compression of the nerves—it's the rare patient with diabetes whose nerve damage is limited to just the feet. Among my patients who have foot neuropathy, about half of them also complain of numbness, tingling, and other symptoms in their hands.

Remember, in 1973, when McComas and Upton discussed the connection between CTS and diabetes, the risk was 16 percent. It isn't coincidental that this is also the time when high-fructose corn syrup was being widely infused into our food supplies. This serves as an example of how metabolic abnormalities that come with high blood sugar can cause problems long before diabetes shows up.

In severe cases, carpal tunnel syndrome is treated with nerve decompression surgery. The pressure on the nerve is released by cutting through the carpal ligament to open up the roof of the tunnel. In 1950, the medical literature reported only *twelve* instances of this operative procedure. And yet, the *New York Times* reports that currently more than 500,000 carpal tunnel procedures are performed every year in the United States. Prevailing medical opinion attributes this radical increase to the introduction of the personal (microcomputer) in 1977. I believe the answer lies elsewhere—with the introduction in 1957 of high-fructose corn syrup. Thus, patients were developing CTS not from typing at a keyboard, but from sipping the soda sitting on the desk. Carpal tunnel syndrome is yet another painful and disabling condition that is largely avoidable just by cutting sugar from your diet.

4. **Do you often have a runny nose, sinus headaches, or need to take over-the-counter or prescription antihistamines (drugs such as Allegra and Claritin)? Have you been diagnosed with chronic sinusitis?**

Sinusitis is an inflammation or infection of the sinuses, the hollow spaces within the skull surrounding the nose. Every year, 30 million cases are diagnosed. Symptoms include headaches, a thick nasal discharge, and often a decreased sense of smell. It's usually acute, meaning it comes on quickly and goes away by itself within a couple of weeks. Most cases of acute sinusitis are caused by having a cold or a respiratory allergy. Sometimes sinusitis can become chronic, meaning it goes on forever, or so it seems.*

You have chronic sinusitis if you've got symptoms for more than a few weeks, or if they go away and come back, or if they just don't ever really go away at all. Generally speaking, constant inflammation causes thickened mucus membranes in the nose and sinus cavities.

Sinusitis is one of the many *itises* that can be traced back to a diet high in sugar. Excess sugar in your body not only ends up in fat cells, but also gets excreted in other ways, such as through your mucus. Your sinuses are a perfect guesthouse for pathogens: They're moist, dark, and warm. And if your diet is crummy, the mucus in them is full of the nutrient

---

Allergic rhinitis (runny nose, sneezing, itchy eyes, congestion) is caused by an allergic reaction to something inhaled, such as pollen, mold, or pet dander. An allergy by definition happens when your immune system, for unknown reasons, overreacts to something and leaps into action. Allergic rhinitis is extremely common—about one in five people has it. As part of the allergic response, your body releases inflammatory substances called histamines. Antihistamines counter the response and dry up your nose.

bacteria love most: sugar. Any bacteria that find their way to your sinuses may decide to settle in for a nice, long stay.

They're hard to evict, because a diet high in sugar also affects your immune system's ability to work efficiently. Stick with me as I explain. The white blood cells that make up your body's immune system need plenty of vitamin C to be at their most effective. In fact, white blood cells may contain as much as 20 times the vitamin C as other types of cells. If you have high blood sugar, however, your cells have trouble absorbing vitamin C, because glucose molecules and vitamin C molecules are very similar in shape.*

In humans, insulin carries both glucose and vitamin C into our cells. But if glucose levels in the blood are too high, the glucose competes with the vitamin C to get in. Glucose always wins, because the insulin receptors in the cell wall have a higher affinity for glucose than for vitamin C. If your blood is awash with excess glucose, vitamin C is the loser.

Let's combine what we know about the competition between glucose and vitamin C with an interesting fact about white blood cells: because they need so much vitamin C to be effective, they have about 50 times as many insulin receptors as other cells.

Now let's connect the dots. If your blood sugar is too high, the white blood cells of your immune system can't get enough vitamin C to work as well as they should. You're much more likely to get sick—and stay sick—with stubborn infections. Ditto for allergic rhinitis. You can't prevent

---

*In fact, in just about all mammals vitamin C is manufactured from glucose in the liver. Humans and other primates, guinea pigs, and fruit bats are the only mammals that can't make their own vitamin C and need to get it from food instead.

allergies, but you can improve how efficiently your immune system responds.

A common self-help recommendation for sinusitis and allergic rhinitis is to take vitamin C supplements. This may help a bit by forcing some extra vitamin C into your cells, but it's approaching the problem from the wrong direction. Cut the sugar from your diet and you will boost your immune system by letting it get all the vitamin C you need—without fighting sugar for the territory.

5. Do you feel tired most or all of the time?

Of all the complaints doctors hear, feeling *tired all the time* is in the top five. In fact, TATT is a common abbreviation in medical charts. Many, many health issues can make you feel tired, of course. If TATT is in your chart, I urge you to work with your doctor to look at possible causes and rule out serious illness, such as cancer or heart disease.

As part of the process, your doctor will order a blood test to check your blood sugar level. Chances are good that if you're tired all the time, your blood sugar will be higher than normal—and you have hyperglycemia. Technically, you're hyperglycemic if your fasting blood sugar is 126 mg/dL, or in the diabetic range. Hyperglycemia doesn't really cause noticeable symptoms, however, until your blood glucose is "astronomical," generally 200 mg/dL or higher.*

Feeling tired all the time is a very common symptom of hyperglycemia; other symptoms include excessive thirst and frequent urination. The cells of your body are desperate for

---

*In fact, having blood sugar of 200 mg/dL or higher at any point, even soon after a meal when blood sugar normally goes up, means you definitely have diabetes.

some glucose, but they have become so resistant to the effects of insulin that the glucose just can't get in. It builds up in your bloodstream instead. You feel fatigued both because your cells can't get any fuel and because the excess glucose in your blood is making the blood thicker than normal. Think of stirring several spoonfuls of sugar into a cup of water. The sugar dissolves and the water becomes a bit syrupy. That's what's happening in your blood. Thick, sludgy blood doesn't circulate very well, so your cells also aren't getting enough oxygen or other nutrients, and their waste products aren't being carried away very efficiently. No wonder you're tired all the time!

By the time the constant fatigue of hyperglycemia sets in, your blood sugar has been slowly creeping up for years. As your blood sugar has been rising, your energy level has been sinking—just so gradually that you didn't really notice. If you meet the definition of the metabolic syndrome in question 1, you may well have tipped over into type 2 diabetes without knowing it. You're not alone—some 19 million Americans have undiagnosed type 2 diabetes.

Over those years of rising blood sugar, you've already done a lot of damage to your nerves. Once your blood sugar rises to seriously hyperglycemic levels, the damage can go quickly from something you didn't even feel to something that's painful and debilitating. You might have neuropathy in one or both feet. In some cases, undiagnosed high blood sugar can lead to *diabetic focal neuropathy*, or neuropathy that suddenly attacks specific nerves in the head, torso, or leg. The most common symptoms are pain and muscle weakness. Depending on the affected nerve, you might also get double vision, Bell's palsy, severe lower back or leg pain, and chest pain that might even be mistaken for a heart attack.

If your blood sugar is high, it's obvious that sugar in the diet is causing your constant fatigue. The solution is also obvious: no more sugar! My patients who eliminate sugar entirely report dramatic changes in their energy levels.

6. **Did you have severe acne in your teen years or do you have adult acne (more than the occasional blemish) now?**

Ask any dermatologist about the link between sugar in the diet and acne and you'll be told emphatically that diet has nothing to do with it. In my mind, this flat-out refusal to even consider diet is a perfect example of how blind the medical profession can be. The evidence that sugar is behind almost all cases of acne is very convincing—and has been published in well-respected medical journals.

Exactly how sugar gives you pimples is a bit complicated, so again, stick with me. You know that when you eat carbohydrates, especially junky refined carbs, your blood sugar jumps and your body produces extra insulin to carry away the glucose. Insulin doesn't just handle glucose, however—and one of its many other functions is to trigger the production of hormones, including one called *insulin-like growth factor 1* (IGF-1). What does IGF-1 do? Among other things, it stimulates production of *sebum*, an oily substance produced by sebaceous glands in the skin. Sebum lubricates and waterproofs your skin and hair; every hair follicle on your skin has at least one sebaceous gland. At the same time, IGF-1 stimulates the growth of skin cells in general, including in the hair follicles. Another hormone stimulated by insulin, insulin-like growth factor binding protein 3 (IGFB-3), makes dead skin cells (which are now occurring faster because of higher insulin levels leading to higher IGF-1 levels) clump together.

High insulin from too much sugar in the diet stimulates the production of sebum; faster growth of skin cells in the hair follicles means more dead cells being shed; IGFB-3 makes those dead cells clump together. You've now got the recipe for a clogged hair follicle, better known as a zit.

On top of all that, male adolescents normally become slightly insulin resistant as they grow toward maturity. That means they produce more insulin, which in turn means they produce more IGF-I—which means they get more zits. And who drinks the most sugar-sweetened sodas (five cans a day is not uncommon), eats the most candy bars, and has the highest consumption of junk food? Male adolescents. It's no surprise that acne is such a problem for them.

The good news about acne is that you don't need expensive and dangerous medications such as Accutane (isotretinoin) to treat it. You don't even need to slather on expensive lotions, creams, and other skin treatments. All you need to do is cut the sugar from your diet. In particular, cut the sugar from crappy junk foods.* Of course, not all acne is caused by excess sugar, although I would argue that a majority is. Consult your dermatologist for a more definitive diagnosis.

7. Do your feet sometimes feel itchy, burning, tingling, or numb?

If you're having itchiness, burning, tingling, or numbness in your feet, you're experiencing the early symptoms of diabetic peripheral neuropathy, which I will discuss in detail in the next chapter. But if you haven't yet been diagnosed

---

*Even the processed vegetable oils in these foods are high in pro-inflammatory omega-6 fatty acids, which only make acne worse.

with type 2 diabetes, you're about to be—at least, that is, if you come to my office.

The unpleasant symptoms of peripheral neuropathy occur when the nerves in your feet are damaged from too much sugar in your bloodstream. It's that simple, really. The nerves have swollen from excess sugar, and these swollen nerves are now pressing up against the surrounding muscle, bone, and connective tissue in your feet. The result is compression—where nerves are being squashed in place and can no longer send and receive impulses normally. Instead, there's static on the line, in the form of pain, tingling, itchiness, and numbness.

If you have diabetes, you are almost certain to get some form of neuropathy—at least 60 to 70 percent probability. The longer you have diabetes, the more certain neuropathy becomes. Almost everyone who has had diabetes for twenty-five years or more will also have neuropathy. Sustained high blood sugar causes neuropathy. Removing sugar from the diet and getting blood sugar under control will go a long way toward ending neuropathy. It's that simple.

8. **Have you ever had gingivitis, periodontal disease, or a root canal?**

I've had extensive conversations with dentists about the reasons for a root canal—the procedure used to repair and salvage an infected, badly decayed, or physically damaged tooth. In the procedure, the nerve and pulp within the root canal cavity of the tooth are removed. The cavity is cleaned out and then filled with a rubber compound called *gutta-percha*. The opening into the cavity is sealed with a filling. The dentists I talk to are convinced that the need for a root canal is caused by a mechanical problem—a hole or crack in the tooth has let infection-causing bacteria into the cavity. I'm not convinced.

I believe this is yet another example of the global compression theory. A high-sugar diet causes a compression of the nerve that supplies the tooth from the trigeminal nerve branch. With compression, the nerve begins to die, just as in diabetic neuropathy. The dentists' hypothesis is that the damage is infection induced, but I contend that it is trauma against the already inflamed trigeminal nerve that leads to the need for a root canal. Millions of root canals are done each year in the United States. This is yet another example of a common nerve problem that is really the result of a compression neuropathy.

9. Do you have skin tags or dark, velvety areas on your skin?

Two very common but often overlooked warning signs of insulin resistance, the metabolic syndrome, and diabetes are skin tags (*achrocordons*) and *acanthosis nigricans*, dark, velvety patches on the skin.

Skin tags are benign growths and often look a little like tiny balloons. They occur most commonly on the neck and in the armpits, but they can also occur on the eyelids, in the genital area, and under the breasts. They're a bit unsightly and can be annoying, but they're harmless. In fact, they're very common—about half of all adults have a few. The real problem with skin tags is that they occur much more often and in greater numbers in overweight people. When that happens, it's a pretty good sign that insulin resistance is also occurring—because high insulin levels stimulate the growth of excess skin cells. Whenever I see a new patient and note multiple skin tags, I know without even looking at the chart that the patient has diabetes.

The same is true for *acanthosis nigricans* (AN), a skin condition causing areas of dark, velvety skin in body folds and creases. It's most commonly seen in the armpits, neck area, and groin. AN is an even more certain sign of diabetes than skin tags. The skin changes are almost always found only in people who are obese or who have diabetes—and the heavier you are, the greater your risk. Like skin tags, acanthosis nigricans is harmless and doesn't require treatment. And like skin tags, it's caused by insulin resistance. Here, too, high insulin levels stimulate abnormal skin growth. What I find most disturbing about AN is that when it happens in an overweight kid, it's a pretty sure predictor of type 2 diabetes at an early age, possibly as soon as the late teens.

I can't say that cutting sugar from your diet will keep you from getting skin tags or AN or make them go away once they occur, but eliminating sugar will likely keep both conditions from getting worse.

10. Are your legs sometimes restless at night (a crawling or creeping sensation relieved by moving)?

That horrible throbbing, creeping, crawling, pulling sensation in your legs at night (or even when you're just sitting quietly) is known as restless legs syndrome (RLS). The sensations create a powerful urge to move your legs to relieve the discomfort. Because RLS occurs at night and may even worsen as the night goes on, it's a major cause of insomnia, daytime sleepiness, and all the bad symptoms of sleep deprivation—including elevated blood sugar. It's considered a sleep disorder, not a complication of diabetes, but that's what it really is for my patients.

Restless legs syndrome is still a medical mystery—we don't know exactly what causes it and why it sometimes goes away for long periods. What we do know is that people with peripheral neuropathy also often get RLS. We also know that people with diabetes are far more likely to have RLS, whether or not they also have peripheral neuropathy—in other words, having diabetes is an independent risk factor for RLS. By some estimates, about 18 percent of people with diabetes have RLS, compared to about 5 percent of people without diabetes. For reasons we still don't understand, women with diabetes are about twice as likely to develop RLS as are men with diabetes.

The sleep disruption of RLS can raise your blood sugar all on its own. If you have RLS and diabetes, the sleep disruption will only make your blood sugar problem even worse. So, getting your blood sugar under control will probably help relieve the RLS symptoms, and relieving the RLS symptoms will help improve your blood sugar. This is good win-win example of how giving up the sugar improves your health.

11. Have you ever had a gallbladder attack or had your gallbladder removed?

Your gallbladder is a small organ that stores bile made in your liver until it's needed for digestion. When bile is needed, your gallbladder pumps it out through a duct leading into the small intestine. Gallstones are hard deposits that form inside the gallbladder. They're very common—at least 20 million adults in the United States have them, though most will never know it. Gallstones are usually quite small, often no larger than a grain of sand, so if one does happen to get pumped out, it passes through the bile duct without any trouble. Sometimes, however, a gallstone can be large enough to get stuck inside the duct, and when that happens, you have a gallbladder attack.* Why do some people with gallstones never even know it, while others end up in the operating room? For many, it's sugar.

People who are overweight or obese are more prone to gallstones. So are people with diabetes. Peter J. Dyck, of the Mayo Clinic in Rochester, Minnesota, is one of the leading neurologists in the country and author of a seminal two-volume textbook, *Peripheral Neuropathy*. Peter Dyck dominates the neurology literature and thinking in the medical world. It is the gold standard for the accepted treatment of diabetic peripheral neuropathy, an "incurable" disease. Dyck points out that 50 percent of people who get gallbladder disease go on to get diabetes. This is an astonishingly high statistic. And when someone with diabetes has a gallbladder attack, the attack is more likely to be severe and lead to an infection.

What's going on here? Two things, both related to sugar. First, a diet high in refined carbohydrates raises your triglycerides—those tiny fat droplets in your bloodstream. High triglycerides seem to encourage the formation of gallstones (we're not sure why), which raises your risk for a gallbladder attack. Second, damage to the nerves that control the gallbladder keeps the organ from contracting as well as it

---

*If you've ever had one, you know a gallbladder attack is very painful—not something you'd ever want to have again. And because if you've had one gallbladder attack, you have a 70 percent chance of having another, most people who develop gallbladder trouble choose to have the organ surgically removed. Cholecystectomy, as the procedure is known, is one of the most common operations in the United States—about half a million are done each year.

should, which means bile doesn't get squirted out efficiently. Every time your gallbladder contracts, some bile remains backed up in it, where it can become sludgy and form gallstones. Then, because the nerve damage keeps the gallbladder from contracting well, the stones that do form are more likely to get stuck in the bile duct instead of being passed out of it into the small intestine.

The type of nerve damage that causes gallbladder attacks is called *autonomic neuropathy*. Autonomic nerves are nerves that operate in the background, automatically sending messages from your brain and spinal cord to your heart, digestive system, bladder, genitals, blood vessels, sweat glands, and the pupils in your eyes. The autonomic nerves take care of everyday housekeeping in your body, controlling everything from your bowels to your heart rate and blood pressure. You never notice the work your autonomic nerves do until something goes wrong. Even then, you don't notice a problem with the nerve itself. Instead, when an autonomic nerve is damaged, the harm shows up in the organ it controls. Autonomic nerves are the first nerves to be affected in the metabolic syndrome process. Autonomic neuropathy is the first stage of peripheral neuropathy and has exactly the same cause: sugar. Eliminating sugar from the diet and getting your blood sugar under control may improve the symptoms of autonomic neuropathy (especially digestive symptoms) and keep them from getting worse. Unfortunately, however, the damage can't be reversed.

Diabetic autonomic neuropathy occurs when these nerves are damaged and can no longer function correctly. It's a very common complication of type 2 diabetes, but the damage begins long before you reach that diagnosis. Years of high blood sugar gradually restrict the blood flow to the nerves, slowly damaging them and eventually impairing their ability to transmit impulses correctly. The sugar itself makes the nerves swell up and stop working well; advanced glycation end products gum it up.

Because the symptoms of diabetic autonomic neuropathy develop slowly, it's only when the nerve damage is fairly far along that you start to notice them. When the autonomic nerves that control your heart are damaged, for instance, your heart might develop an abnormal beat or rhythm, with possible fatal consequences. When the autonomic nerves that control your digestive system are damaged, you get gallbladder attacks, problems with constipation and diarrhea, nausea after eating, and a range of other unpleasant symptoms.

12. Do you have frequent (more than two times a week) heartburn, upset stomach, constipation, or diarrhea?

Frequent digestive problems can have a wide range of causes, yet in my experience the most common cause, sugar, is often overlooked. Years of high blood sugar, starting long before diabetes is diagnosed, damage the autonomic nerves that control your digestive system from end to end. Eventually, like nearly 75 percent of all people with diabetes, you develop some form of diabetic autonomic neuropathy. For example, nearly half of all people with diabetes have at least some signs of *gastroparesis*, or partial paralysis of the stomach muscles caused by damage to the vagus nerve. Gastroparesis keeps your stomach from emptying its contents into your small intestine normally, leading to a variety of unpleasant symptoms, including severe heartburn, bloating, nausea, vomiting, dangerous blood sugar swings, and the aptly named dumping syndrome.

Many of my patients have been scoped and scanned up

and down in an attempt to find the source of their ongoing digestive issues, only to be told that the problem must be
stress. That's doctor-speak for "I have no idea what's wrong
with you, so I'm blaming it on your mental issues. Take these
antidepressants and these antacids and come back in three
months."

The doctors are only trying to help their patients, of
course, but if the problems are caused by autonomic neuropathy, these drugs will actually make them worse. Once again,
let's connect some dots. Diabetic autonomic neuropathy is
caused by nerve damage from sugar. The most commonly
prescribed antidepressants today are selective serotonin reuptake inhibitors (SSRIs) such as Lexapro (escitalopram),
Prozac (fluoxetine), Paxil (paroxetine), and Zoloft (sertraline).
While these drugs may help relieve symptoms of depression,
they also raise your blood sugar and increase your risk of
type 2 diabetes.

About a quarter of all people who take these drugs will
also gain weight—not good for the blood sugar or for nerves
that are already damaged. Antacids, especially proton pump
inhibitors (PPIs) such as Prilosec (omeprazole), Prevacid (lan-
soprazole), Nexium (esomeprazole), and Protonix (pantopra-
zole), can block your absorption of vitamin B_{12} (crucial for
healthy nerves) and lower your levels of magnesium. (Many
people with diabetes are low on this essential mineral.) This
is also not good for nerves that are already damaged. Put the
two drug classes together and, while there may be some temporary relief of symptoms, in the end the combination only
worsens the neuropathy.

Unfortunately, there's not a lot we can do to reverse autonomic neuropathy once it starts. Getting the blood sugar
under control by removing sugar from the diet usually helps

to slow down or even halt the neuropathy. And if the problem is caught early enough, lifestyle changes and standard treatments can help quite a bit with the symptoms.

13. Do you get frequent (more than once a year) bladder or yeast infections?

Bladder infections, also known as urinary tract infections (UTIs) or *cystitis*, are very common among women—nearly half of all women have had a bladder infection at some point.*
If you get them frequently, however, you probably have high blood sugar, even if you don't know it yet. The excess glucose in your bloodstream is making you much more susceptible to UTIs both directly and indirectly.

Directly, excess sugar from your bloodstream is excreted through your kidneys and ends up in your urine. In fact, one of the oldest diagnostic tests in medical history is tasting the urine. If it tasted sweet, the patient had diabetes. Sugary urine is a fertile breeding ground for bacteria, which is why women with diabetes are two to three times more likely to have bacteria in their bladder than are women without diabetes. At any given time, about 20 percent of all women with diabetes have a bladder infection.

Indirectly, you're getting UTIs because the excess sugar in your blood has slowly damaged the autonomic nerves controlling your bladder. More than half of all people with diabetes have some degree of damage to the nerves that control the bladder. Among other things, the nerve damage means you'll have trouble emptying your bladder fully. The leftover urine pooling in the bladder makes a great place for bacteria to breed. At the same time, diabetes also causes poor circulation to the

---

*Men do get bladder infections, but far less often.

area, which limits how many white blood cells can arrive to fight the infection; high blood sugar limits how well the white blood cells work. It's not surprising that women with diabetes are more likely to end up in the hospital from a UTI.

If you get frequent bladder infections, even if your blood sugar is normal, eliminating sugar from your diet will almost certainly help cut back on them. You'll get the infections less often, the symptoms will be less annoying, and you'll get over them faster.

What goes for UTIs also goes for yeast infections, also known as *candidiasis*. Vaginal yeast infections are very common among all women, but women with type 2 diabetes get them a lot more often. If your blood sugar is consistently high, even if you don't have diabetes, the mucus in your vagina will contain excess sugar, just as your urine will. Single-celled yeast organisms are normally found in the vagina in small numbers. Take that moist, warm environment and add sugar to it, and the yeast take off, multiplying rapidly and causing unpleasant symptoms such as a thick white discharge, itching, and burning during urination. As with the bladder, over the long run high blood sugar reduces blood circulation to the area, which makes it that much harder for your white blood cells to get to the infection and fight it off.

Getting your blood sugar under control is an essential first step in treating and preventing yeast infections.

Past Problems Predict Present Problems

Wendy, in her late forties, came to my office seeking relief for her achy, burning feet. She reported taking two common drugs for high blood pressure, and was overweight, but the standard medical history revealed no other health issues.

I asked about the high blood pressure.

She responded, "I don't have high blood pressure because I take medicine to keep it down."

I explained there's a difference between the normal numbers she had when I took her blood pressure and having the disease called high blood pressure, but she didn't want to think of herself as someone with a chronic disease. I knew she wasn't going to like what I'd have to say after checking her feet.

Her foot discomfort was caused by the earliest phase of diabetic peripheral neuropathy. A lifetime of eating sugar had caught up to her—causing mild damage to the small nerves in her feet and resulting in some numbness. Fortunately, the damage hadn't progressed too far and she could quickly reverse by cutting sugar from her diet.

Wendy had different ideas.

"My family doctor checked my blood sugar and said it was just a little on the high side," she said. "How can I have diabetic neuropathy if I don't have diabetes?"

I explained that the actual number doesn't matter. Her fasting blood sugar was 112 mg/dL—below 125 mg/dL, the official level for diabetes as recognized by the American Diabetes Association—but she was still in trouble because it's the long-term trend that counts. She already had three out of the five markers for the metabolic syndrome: high blood sugar, excess weight in the stomach area, and high blood pressure.

Next stop on the blood sugar express: type 2 diabetes.

"Did you have acne as a teenager?" I asked.

"Yes," she said. "It was awful. It didn't clear up until I went to college."

"Let me guess," I said. "You became a vegetarian then, right?"

"I did! I told everyone I didn't want to eat anything that had a mother because it made me seem cool, but it was really so I could lose weight. It worked, too. Instead of gaining the freshman fifteen, I lost it. Of course, I've gained it back and more since then. How did you know that?"

"Because when you became a vegetarian to lose weight you stopped eating junk food, too. With sugar out of your diet, your skin cleared up. Now, let me make another guess. You've always suffered with headaches."

"And they're getting worse," she said. "When I was young, I had migraines."

"Your body has never handled sugar very well—that's why you got acne and migraines and it's why you get headaches now. It's also why you're having foot trouble and high blood sugar. We can stop your foot neuropathy and keep you from getting diabetes, but it means big changes."

Wendy was still unconvinced. What she wanted was a magic pill to make her foot pain go away; instead I gave her advice on taking care of her feet and keeping an eye out for anything that looked like a cut or infection. I also gave her a diet plan and scheduled her for follow-up in three months.

A few weeks later, I was surprised to see her again. Wendy was there because her kitten had scratched her on the foot. She hadn't even noticed at first, but in a few days that tiny scratch had become an infected, painful sore that kept getting worse instead of healing naturally.

I decided to lay it all on the line.

"You have some numbness in your foot, so you didn't notice the scratch. Bacteria got into your skin and your high blood sugar fed them the food they like best. Now you have a real problem that's going to take weeks of antibiotics and bandages to get better. And this is just the start. I guarantee that you'll be back with another infection within a year. And ten years down the line, I could be cutting off your foot. The choice is pretty simple: change your diet or lose your foot."

She was finally listening. There's nothing like a painful hole in your foot and the threat of amputation to get your attention.

"I guess I really do need to eat better," she said. "Can I have that diet again?"

Because she decided to remove sugar and junk carbohydrates from her diet, Wendy's foot healed a bit faster than I expected. I'm happy to say her neuropathy also improved quite a bit, to the point where I no longer need to see her.

6

The Five Phases
of Peripheral Neuropathy

HEED THE CLARION CALL

Years ago a patient sat in my office and told me he just couldn't "cowboy" anymore. He worked the oldest ranch in Arizona—some five thousand acres of grassland, dry gullies, and cattle. A cattleman steers his horse with his legs and feet—he braces in the stirrup and automatically communicates quick shifts in direction or momentum as together they tend the stock. Deep into stage 4 peripheral neuropathy, my patient could no longer "feel" the ride and he was afraid the life he loved was over.

Neuropathy is a slow, insidious process. It takes years of a diet high in sugar (including grain-based carbohydrates and alcohol)* to damage your nerves enough to feel the

---

*Alcoholic neuropathy comes as the result of long-term and sustained use. Usually, nerve damage is irreversible and while a patient with alcoholism most likely dies from other causes (such as liver failure, cardiovascular disease, and "nonnatural/social" events), alcoholic neuropathy severely affects quality of life.

earliest symptoms. The longer you go on with high blood sugar and eventually diabetes, the more likely you are to develop neuropathy. When they're first diagnosed, about 8 percent of people with type 2 diabetes also already have neuropathy. After twenty-five years with the disease, at least half will have neuropathy to some degree, and over a lifetime with diabetes, the odds of impairment are practically 100 percent.

Every day, I see patients who are severely limited by peripheral neuropathy in their feet. They're in pain, they have foot ulcers that won't heal, and they're using canes, crutches, walkers, even wheelchairs. Some have had more than one amputation and are missing toes, feet, and parts of their legs.

If you're at high risk or have already been diagnosed with metabolic syndrome, prediabetes, or type 2 diabetes, you almost certainly already have peripheral neuropathy. You just don't know it yet. You're probably dismissing the way your feet feel tired all the time by telling yourself you've been on them a lot. The same is true for burning and aching sensations in your feet, your sweaty toes, and those foot and leg cramps you get at night.

Stop fooling yourself. What you're feeling in your feet isn't normal. These sensations are the first hints of peripheral neuropathy and big trouble to come.

As for the cowboy, eventually, I operated on him and now he's back in the saddle.

Symptoms of Pain and Numbness

Let's talk about the pain and numbness caused by neuropathy. It comes in a lot of different forms, all of them unpleasant. Most people with early stage neuropathy experience fo discomfort in one or more of the following ways:

- Burning sensation
- Tired or achy feet
- Itchiness
- Tingling or pins-and-needles sensation
- Sudden, painful electric shock sensation
- Muscle spasms or cramps
- Extreme sensitivity to cold or heat
- Extreme sensitivity to touch
- Restless legs syndrome
- Formication (the sensation of having ants or other small insects crawling over your skin)

Understanding the Phases

Knowing what phase of neuropathy you're in is crucial to treating it correctly and possibly reversing it. Much more important, knowing what phase you're in can help prevent further complications. The more severe your foot neuropathy, the greater your risk of amputation.

Based on my experience, I classify foot neuropathy into five phases of increasing severity:

- Phase 1: Intermittent pain and numbness
- Phase 2: Intermittent pain and numbness; over time the pain and numbness become more frequent and intense
- Phase 3: Constant pain, usually on medication, trouble sleeping due to discomfort

ments of pain relief, less pain, more numbness
pain, all numbness

what phase you're in, and no matter whether you've been diagnosed with diabetes or not, your neuropathy is the result of a diet that's full of sugar.

Phase 1: Intermittent Pain and Numbness— Blood Sugar Reads Normal

In phase 1, symptoms are intermittent—you may go hours, days, or even months without feeling any discomfort. When you do feel the symptoms, they tend to be more painful or evident at night.

The numbness caused by phase 1 foot neuropathy is subtle. The sensation is sort of like wearing a very thin stocking. At first, you might not even notice it, but I can tell right away by testing your ankle reflexes with my little hammer. As foot numbness progresses, you will have trouble keeping your balance when you walk. Down the line, you'll need a cane or walker to keep from falling.

If you're having phase 1 neuropathy, you've probably come directly to me rather than being referred by your primary care physician. Although your symptoms are being caused by sugar in your diet, at this stage you probably haven't been diagnosed with type 2 diabetes. You've come to me because your feet hurt.

In fact, if you have phase 1 neuropathy, your fasting blood sugar is probably normal. The illness is in the earliest stage and your pancreas is still functioning. However, to get a clearer picture of the damage already occurring in your body at this early stage, it is important to do a *fasting serum insulin test*, which measures the amount of insulin in your blood, not the amount of glucose, after a twelve-hour fast. If your fasting serum insulin levels are elevated (over 5 mcU/mL),* you are showing the earliest stages of the full-blown diabetes to come. Many agree that keeping your fasting serum insulin level under 3 is healthiest.

Phase 1 neuropathy can be halted in its tracks and easily reversed—if you are willing to eliminate all sugar, wheat, and processed foods, as well as add a better balance of dietary fats. This is the *only* certain way to stop the neuropathy now. As the phases progress, neuropathy becomes increasingly difficult to treat—and increasingly dangerous.

Phase 2: More Frequent Pain and Numbness

In phase 2, the pain and numbness are still intermittent but becoming more frequent and intense. Your nerves are being damaged a bit more each day by your high blood sugar. You might be seeing me now because your doctor has finally diagnosed your blood sugar issues, or you might already be my patient but you haven't heeded my warnings. No matter what, you're reaching a tipping point. Change your diet now, or move on to the later, more painful, and more dangerous phases of neuropathy.

Phase 3: Drugs—and Complications

When you reach phase 3 of peripheral neuropathy, you have almost certainly been formally diagnosed with type 2 diabetes, probably by your primary care doctor, but possibly by me. You're now in constant pain.

Paradoxically, your feet also feel more numb, so you're less steady when you stand up and walk. At this point, many

*Micro unit per milliliter.

of my patients are taking powerful drugs such as *pregabalin* (marketed as Lyrica) to help them deal with the unending pain. These drugs provide some symptom relief, at the price of drowsiness, dizziness, and other nasty side effects, including suicidal thoughts. None of these side effects will do much for getting you back to a normal life.*

At this phase, you are now much more likely to develop a diabetic ulcer on the bottom of your foot (called a plantar ulcer). This begins as a minor injury to the skin—perhaps nothing more than a scratch from stepping barefoot on something—but because you can't really feel your feet very well anymore, you don't notice you've hurt yourself. Ordinarily, that wouldn't really matter. Your immune system would take over and heal up the damage.

However, your body isn't ordinary anymore. By now you have extensive damage to the small nerve fibers of your feet. When the small fibers are that damaged, the blood circulation to the skin of your feet is affected as well. Because the blood flow to the skin is now abnormal, that small scratch that you didn't feel can't heal properly. Infection-fighting white blood cells don't get through, and the area can't get enough oxygen and other nutrients to grow new cells. What happens then? A minor injury turns into a big, painful, hard-to-heal hole in your foot. In the worst-case scenario, that hole becomes gangrenous. Today, we can do a lot to heal a gangrenous foot and avoid amputation, but chopping off a toe or two or even your whole foot is still a real possibility.

Diabetic foot ulcers are just miserable to suffer through. The treatment is long, slow, painful—and very expensive. You'll miss many days of work; you'll need a lot of appoint-

*More in Chapter 7.

ments with me; you'll need expensive prescriptions, and you may end up in the emergency room or the hospital. About a quarter of all people with diabetes will develop at least one foot ulcer. The total cost for treating them each year in the United States runs as high as $13 billion.

The long-term results can be more dire. If you have foot ulcers, your risk of premature death from any cause is almost doubled. Your chances of a fatal heart attack are more than twice that of someone without an ulcer; your risk of a fatal stroke jumps about 40 percent. And, of course, there's the risk of *sepsis*, or severe blood infection, originating in the ulcer. Sepsis can lead to organ failure and death.

Getting your glucose under control at this phase is no longer a choice—it's a matter of life or death. As your peripheral foot neuropathy worsens, so does your risk of other dangerous complications from diabetes. This is your last chance to do something to stop the process. Once you pass phase 3, most of the damage to your nerves can't be reversed.

Phase 4: Less Pain, More Risk

By the time you reach phase 4, you might think your foot neuropathy is improving, because it doesn't hurt as much. It isn't. These moments of pain relief are actually because you're developing numbness. Your nerves are slowly disintegrating and losing their ability to transmit information. And so in addition to damage to the small nerve fibers in your feet, you now have damage to the larger fibers as well. And because it is large nerve fibers that help you sense touch and vibration as well as *proprioception* (knowing where your feet are), damage to them makes your feet feel even more numb. At this point, you've become increasingly disabled. Walking can be difficult as your sense of balance is practically nonexistent. You are susceptible to falls and ancillary injury. You're probably also experiencing at least one other disabling complication of diabetes, such as autonomic neuropathy,* and you may well be experiencing heart disease, kidney problems, and vision problems from diabetic retinopathy. You may now be injecting insulin along with taking an array of drugs to control your high blood pressure, cholesterol, and pain.

By this stage, you've done a great deal of damage to all your nerves. Not all of it can be reversed, but eliminating sugar from your diet will still help improve the peripheral neuropathy in your feet.

Phase 5: Feeling No Pain
(Because You've Lost All Sensation)

Sometimes a long-term patient will tell me, "Doctor, the pain is gone! My feet must be getting better." It hurts to tell her that the exact opposite is true. She's no longer in pain because she's lost all sensation in her feet—the hallmark of progression to phase 5. Now the risk of dangerous infection, bad falls, and amputation is higher than ever. Even worse, the chance to help her nerves heal by changing her diet and controlling her diabetes is long past. But there is still hope for these patients, as I'll discuss in the next chapter.

How Clinical Tests Can Confirm
Early Stages of Neuropathy

Your feet hurt and you've come to me to find out why. The last thing you want to hear is that this is just the beginning

---

*Autonomic neuropathy disrupts signals between your brain and the autonomic nervous system that affects involuntary body functions: heart rate, blood pressure, perspiration, and digestion.

of other diseases you're most likely to develop. And yet there are steps to be taken and you should be aware of them as you move forward. First and foremost is to thoroughly review your medical history. Then we can use a number of tests to determine if you have peripheral neuropathy, the specific phase of development, and what you can do about it.

1. A1C. Also called HbA1c or the glycated hemoglobin level. This is a simple blood test to track your blood sugar over a three-month period. Normal range is between 4 and 5.6 percent, meaning the hemoglobin* in your blood has glucose stuck to it. If your A1C is between 5.7 and 6.4 percent, you've got extra glucose and are at risk of developing diabetes. If it's 6.5 percent or higher, you already have the disease.

2. Monofilament test. Also called the Semmes-Weinstein test, this simple procedure uses a piece of nylon wire (resembling a fishing line) that is pressed against areas of your foot so you identify when you can and cannot feel the pressure. When I conduct the test, I focus on the big toe and third toe in each foot, since that's where peripheral neuropathy usually starts. Unfortunately, numbness is a relatively late sign of diabetic neuropathy.†

3. An NCS, or a nerve conductivity study, is the gold standard for determining how your muscles are being affected. Attaching a surface electrode (pad) we can test how quickly electrical impulses are moving through your nerve fibers.

---

*A protein in your red blood cells that carries oxygen to all the places you need it.

†A similar subjective test involves measuring the cutaneous pressure threshold.

4. A PSSD, or a pressure-specified sensory device, is a quantitative sensory test developed by Dellon in conjunction with an engineer from NASA. A two-pronged instrument determines how you detect pressure from two separate contact points. The more damage to your sensory nerves, the farther apart the prongs must be for you to detect them separately.

5. Punch biopsy. With a specialized tool, the doctor takes a tiny core of skin from the top of your foot and your leg. Examined under a microscope, a pathologist can see the small nerve fibers and determine how densely packed they are. Normally you would have many clearly visible nerve fibers; but if you have peripheral neuropathy, some of the nerve fibers have probably started to die and won't be visible. Even if the neuropathy isn't far enough along for nerve fibers to be missing, the staining shows areas of the nerves that are swollen or have other abnormalities. This is very helpful for early diagnosis.

6. The sympathetic skin response (SSR) and the sudomotor scan can also detect early small fiber neuropathy by measuring sweat output in your feet (too much or too little perspiration can also be an early indicator of neuropathy).

7. Once neuropathy has been diagnosed, we need to track it over time to see if you're getting better, staying the same, or getting worse. If your habits don't change and you ignore my clinical observations, your disease will worsen. That will inevitably lead to pain. And lots of it.

7

Meanwhile, Just Make It Stop

WHAT WE SUFFER TO EASE THE PAIN

Imagine it's the middle of the night; you're asleep in your bed and a fire alarm pierces the darkness. You smell smoke and sense overwhelming heat, but you yank the battery out of the alarm and go back to sleep. Does that make sense? Yet it's what you do every time you pop a pill to dull the pain of peripheral neuropathy. Not only are you neglecting to address the source of the problem—you're essentially pouring more fuel on the fire.

In the early phases, peripheral neuropathy might be the only symptom you feel as your blood sugar rises and you gradually move toward the metabolic syndrome and diabetes. Aside from an expanding waistline, early symptoms, such as high blood pressure or high cholesterol, are painless and invisible. Your tired, achy feet, to say nothing of painful pricks and periodic numbness, are the first wisps of smoke as the fire of neuropathy smolders. At this point, you have a clear choice: put out the fire now by changing your diet, or face a raging inferno down the line. Unfortunately, at the later phases of neuropathy, nerve damage to your feet cannot be fully reversed.

Beginning nerve damage is painful. The term for the sharp, prickling sensation first felt is called *formication*, from the Latin *to crawl like an ant* because people describe it as having "biting insects crawling on the skin." This is usually followed with burning sensations, restless legs, and sensitivity to cold, heat, and touch. My patients often tell me that the discomfort is worse at night, keeping them from sleep; and during the day, the pain can be bad enough to keep them housebound. By the time they see me they're often depressed and hopeless—they just want me to do something. Specifically, they want me to prescribe painkilling drugs.

Before reaching for my prescription pad, I ask them, "Why painkillers when that's only part of the solution?" I list the serious drawbacks of these drugs along with their benefits. And, most important, I ask them to work with me in exploring every other option to relieve their pain. The primary goal is not just numbing away pain, but dealing with the underlying problem of uncontrolled blood sugar. If not, I'll be prescribing painkillers for them right up until the time I must cut off their feet—and beyond, as well.

For most of my patients with phase 1 and 2 neuropathy, simply eliminating sugar from the diet does the trick. Within a few weeks, pain improves markedly or even goes away completely. For patients with more advanced neuropathy, improvement from cutting out sugar takes longer to kick in. And for these individuals, pain and numbness improve, but they don't fully subside. Reducing pain is a primary goal, but even if some pain lingers, getting your blood sugar under control sharply reduces your risk of complications from foot neuropathy. And it sharply reduces your development of diabetes with its myriad of severe health issues. These are major accomplishments.

Popular Painkillers and the Power of Big Pharma

To understand why the painkilling drugs usually prescribed for neuropathy can cause more problems than they help, let's look closely at two commonly prescribed medications: Lyrica (pregabalin) and Neurontin (gabapentin).

Both were developed as treatments for individuals with epilepsy that wasn't well controlled with other drugs. That's why they're classified as *anticonvulsants* by the FDA. They're not *opiates*, such as Vicodin or OxyContin, so they're less likely to cause dependence or be abused. Pregabalin and gabapentin seem to activate in your brain by binding to a channel in the central nervous system that controls, among other things, the production of chemicals sending messages back and forth among your cells. If that sounds vague, it is. Despite many theories and research, we still don't know exactly how these drugs work; but that hasn't stopped doctors from prescribing them.

Then, in 2004, Lyrica was approved by the FDA for treating painful diabetic neuropathy; and since has been okayed for many other ailments, including restless legs syndrome, migraines, and fibromyalgia. It's now one of Pfizer's top-selling drugs, with sales of $4.6 billion in 2013. That's a lot of pills.

Chemically, Neurontin is almost identical to Lyrica except that *it costs considerably less and is available as a generic*. However, Neurontin hasn't been FDA approved for

diabetic neuropathy, and because Pfizer also owns Neurontin (having purchased Warner-Lambert in 2000), the com-
pany has no incentive to get the approval. Meanwhile, Lyrica
is locked up in patents until 2019.

Pfizer also ran into legal problems for its marketing practices for Neurontin. Any drug that has been approved for the
FDA to treat a specific condition can be prescribed legally by
a doctor for any other condition; it's known as off-label use.
Although doctors are allowed to do this and often do, drug
companies can only *promote* a drug for its FDA-approved
uses—not for off-label use. That didn't stop the Pfizer sales-
people from promoting Neurontin for off-label uses ranging
from migraines to insomnia, without any studies to back up
their claims. To persuade doctors to prescribe Neurontin,
Pfizer paid leading physicians large sums to present claims
for the drug at lavish dinners and other events, and invited
doctors to attend for free.

Eventually, the FDA caught on and in 2004, Pfizer was
fined the record amount of $430 million for fraudulently
promoting the drug. Did this put much of a dent in the fi-
nances of the world's largest drugmaker? Probably not—that
same year, sales of Neurontin topped $2.7 billion.*

Pfizer got into very big trouble by aggressively promoting Neurontin for conditions that it didn't help. However,
as a treatment for the *pain* of diabetic neuropathy, it does
work—and is far less expensive than Lyrica. Yet my patients
see TV ads for Lyrica and insist on it, not generic gabapentin
or Neurontin.

---

*After all the legal maneuvers, the case was settled in 2014 for $325 mil-
lion.

The Web Becomes Ever More Tangled

In 2011, Lyrica also got a big boost from the American Academy of Neurology (AAN), whose experts issued an official guideline for treating painful diabetic neuropathy that recognized Lyrica as an effective treatment. The guideline was based on a review of the available scientific studies of diabetic nerve treatments. According to the AAN, of all treatments they rated, only Lyrica had "strong evidence" for its effectiveness. Of course, none of the studies the AAN reviewed compared Lyrica to other nondrug treatments, much less dietary changes. With money as the weapon of choice, Big Pharma wins again.

When you start taking anticonvulsant drugs for the pain of peripheral neuropathy, you end up right where Big Pharma wants you: a lifetime consumer of an expensive drug that only masks symptoms and doesn't deal with the underlying cause.

If you're like many of my patients who need to start taking these drugs, you're probably already hooked in a lifetime relationship with at least one other drug. If you have diabetes, for example, you might be taking one of the many different—and expensive—drugs that work by making your cells a little less resistant to insulin, or by forcing your overworked pancreas to squeeze out a bit more insulin. Do they do anything to deal with what actually causes diabetes? No, not at all. In fact, because they make your diabetes seem a bit better, at least as measured by your blood sugar numbers, the people who take them figure that they don't have to do anything else, such as avoiding sugar and becoming more active. Most of these drugs actually make it harder to lose weight, which is step one on the diabetes self-help list. Some raise your risk of having a heart attack, while others can damage your kidneys, and some may increase your risk of deadly pancreatic cancer. These drugs only contribute to the slow, inexorable descent into worsening diabetes and worsening neuropathy.

Recent research has revealed a similar effect from taking statin drugs. Rather than make the most crucial dietary change for lowering your cholesterol—eliminating sugar from the diet—people who take statin drugs tend to gradually start overeating and gaining weight. In fact, over time, people who take statins gain more weight than people who don't. Why? The statin users figure the drug is taking care of their high cholesterol, so they can now eat anything they want. Big Pharma loves this. You're already a lifetime customer for their statin drugs. Soon you'll also be a lifetime customer for their diabetes drugs, their high blood pressure drugs, and their pain drugs, and maybe a couple more. As you get sicker and poorer, Big Pharma gets even richer.

Treating the out-of-control blood sugar that is the underlying cause of peripheral neuropathy is much more effective and cheaper than powerful psychoactive drugs. For patients in the earlier phases of neuropathy, cutting the sugar means an end to the constant assault on their nerves. Pain diminishes or even disappears, and the damaged nerves can repair and even regenerate. Even patients who are at phases 4 and 5 in their neuropathy, where nerve damage is more likely to be permanent, have far less pain when they cut out the sugar. Much more important, at any phase of neuropathy cutting sugar makes a huge difference in the risk of infection and ulceration.

Treating Pain Doesn't Treat the Cause

To call Lyrica (or Neurontin) a treatment for diabetic neuropathy is very misleading. No painkiller, Lyrica included, treats the underlying cause of the neuropathy. All painkillers can do is *relieve* pain and they don't even do that very well. Your feet might temporarily feel better because your brain has been numbed out, but your neuropathy isn't being addressed at all. Unfortunately, as you're now less aware of the pain, you're also *less* motivated to make the dietary changes that could actually save your nerves and keep the neuropathy from getting worse.

Risky Side Effects

Even though my mission is to help you reverse the damage of compression, I don't want anyone to be in pain, so of course I prescribe anticonvulsant drugs when necessary. However, as with many medications, the side effects of anticonvulsants don't simply evaporate—you can be stuck with them. These include:

Sedation and Dizziness

Lyrica and Neurontin make many feel tired, sedated, spaced-out, and dizzy. When I prescribe these drugs, it's usually because the patient is in such pain that she's having trouble sleeping at night. If she avoids daytime use and takes the pill before bedtime, she can use the sleepiness side effect to her advantage and get some rest. When a drug makes you sleepy and spacey during the day, it wrecks your quality of life. Driving, for example, is an especially bad idea. When you feel drowsy all the time and are stuck at home, that makes you sedentary and depressed—which only makes your diabetes worse.

Dizziness is another side effect that is very problematic. If you have serious foot neuropathy, your balance may already be off because your feet are numb, making you feel very unsteady. You might also have poor balance when standing because you have autonomic neuropathy, another likely complication of diabetes, and because you're probably taking at least two different blood pressure medications. A drug that causes dizziness added to already shaky balance is a formula for stumbling and tripping, which can lead to cuts and bruises on the feet, which can lead to ulceration and all its consequences. Dizziness can also cause the sort of nasty fall that leads to a concussion or a broken bone. When older adults break a bone, the complications often lead to surgery, a stay in a nursing home, and a downhill spiral that can end in death. I want everyone to keep mobility and independence, not lose them to drugs.

Swelling in the Hands and Feet

Swollen feet from anticonvulsants are a good example of how a bad situation can be made worse. The last thing someone with peripheral neuropathy needs is a drug that makes his or her feet swell. Already susceptible to damage, swelling of the skin makes it even more vulnerable to damage from shoes that no longer fit, socks that cause blisters, and cuts, scrapes, and bruises. Swelling from Lyrica and Neurontin is more likely if you also take an *angiotensin-converting enzyme* (ACE) inhibitor drug for your blood pressure. ACE inhibitors are the *-pril* drugs, such as Lotensin (benazepril), Capoten (captopril), and Vasotec (enalapril). Many of my patients already take these drugs, which means I rarely prescribe anticonvulsants for them.

Weight Gain

Most people who take Lyrica or Neurontin will gain weight that is impossible to lose while on the drug. This not only worsens diabetes; it's also very discouraging to patients who have worked hard to lose weight and improve blood sugar. The average weight gain is about ten pounds, but some patients gain even more. Diabetes worsens—and so does neuropathy.

Suicidal Thoughts

A well-known side effect of anticonvulsant drugs is suicidal thoughts. Many of my patients are already feeling more than a little depressed and anxious because of their neuropathy. Some of them also have other serious health issues, which naturally contribute to feelings of sadness and worry. It's a terrible idea—especially because these drugs interact badly with Ativan (lorazepam), one of the most commonly prescribed anti-anxiety drugs.

Drug Interactions

Neurontin and Lyrica can cause bad interactions when they're taken with many other drugs. Aside from lorazepam and the swelling caused when they're taken along with ACE inhibitors, these drugs also interact badly with some diabetes medications and narcotic pain medicines. You're much more likely to have serious issues with sleepiness and dizziness when these drugs are combined. In fact, while you're taking anticonvulsants, you should avoid all forms of alcohol, even if it's just an occasional glass of wine with dinner. Just another example of how these drugs can limit your quality of life.

Effectiveness

For all the side effects, risks, and expense, do these drugs really help with the pain? Not completely and often not very much at all. In pain management, a good result would be a 50 percent reduction in pain; an acceptable result would be a 30 percent reduction in pain. Most of my patients see a benefit of some pain reduction, but it rarely approaches 50 percent, even when they take the maximum dose. Some patients are less responsive and stop taking the drug because the side effects are worse than the pain.

Finally, a major concern I have with these drugs is that we don't have enough information on what happens when you take them over the long term.

Other Drugs Used for Neuropathy Pain

Certainly, there are other painkillers. The following critique simply reflects my clinical observations of what does and does not happen within my own protocols and my own patients.

1. At one point, the anticonvulsant drug *topiramate* (Topamax) was used as a treatment for neuropathic pain. It was believed to temporarily work much as other anticonvulsant drugs do; yet for some reason, it just doesn't. While some doctors use it as a last resort, I rarely prescribe this drug.

2. Tricyclic antidepressants such as *nortriptyline* (Aventyl) aren't officially approved by the FDA for neuropathic pain, but they're actually pretty effective. They work well

enough that the International Association for the Study of Pain recommends nortriptyline as a first-line medication for neuropathic pain. The downside is that this drug interacts badly with a long list of other common medications, including some for high blood pressure, diabetes, asthma, and other conditions. So many of my patients have had such unpleasant side effects with this drug that most have stopped taking it. Examples include nausea, drowsiness, nightmares, dry mouth, difficulty urinating, constipation, and loss of interest in sex.

3. The drug *duloxetine* (Cymbalta) is a serotonin-norepinephrine reuptake inhibitor (SNRI). Most commonly used to treat major depression, it's also FDA approved for diabetic peripheral neuropathy. In my experience, this drug is not to be taken lightly. It has a lot of nasty side effects. Like the anticonvulsants, it does nothing to deal with the underlying cause of the neuropathy—it simply masks the pain and doesn't even do that very well. Plus, it's expensive. Side effects include the same drowsiness and dizziness as with Lyrica and Neurontin, as well as nausea, raised blood pressure, dry mouth, decreased appetite, and constipation. Cymbalta interacts badly with a long list of common medications. As with all antidepressants, duloxetine can also affect your sex life, mostly by making you lose interest in it. Not to mention the suicidal thoughts it can cause.

4. *Venlafaxine* (Effexor) works in much the same way as duloxetine. It has all the advantages (none) and all the disadvantages, with one addition—it's risky for people with heart problems.

5. Opioid drugs such as *hydrocodone* (Vicodin) and *oxycodone* (OxyContin, Percocet) are a last resort for treating

neuropathic pain. These drugs, despite their dangers of abuse and dependence, are excellent for relieving many kinds of serious pain and for palliative care. However, the studies show that opioids barely work better than placebos for neuropathy.

6. *Tramadol* (Ultram) is a weak opioid drug that also slows reuptake of serotonin and norepinephrine. This drug is reasonably effective for neuropathic pain relief. It works quickly and it's less likely than the stronger opioids to cause dependence or be abused. On the other hand, it has all the side effects of opioids, including dizziness, sleepiness, nausea, and constipation. Moreover, in August 2014, the FDA made Ultram a Class II narcotic.

7. *Nonsteroidal anti-inflammatory drugs* (NSAIDs) such as over-the-counter aspirin, *acetaminophen* (Tylenol), and *ibuprofen* (Advil) are pretty much useless for chronic peripheral neuropathy, although they may give a little relief during an acute attack. After taking these drugs on their own without results, many patients in the early phases of neuropathy realize they need to come to me. Even prescription NSAIDs such as *naproxen* (Naprosyn) are ineffective, but they have the added disadvantage of upsetting your digestion.

After reading all of this, do you still think that just popping a pill is the solution to peripheral neuropathy? I'm afraid it's not.

Clinical Alternatives to Pill Popping

It may not have a Super Bowl ad, but the treatment that works best for painful diabetic neuropathy is getting your blood sugar under control. Improvement and pain relief don't come overnight, however, and you may have done enough damage to your nerves that you will always have some pain. And yet, in the interim we still have effective ways to relieve pain without handing you a bottle of pills.

Lidocaine Patches

Lidocaine is a safe and effective treatment for painful feet. You've probably had this topical anesthetic at the dentist's office to numb your gum before a Novocain shot. For foot pain, we use prescription stick-on skin patches containing 5 percent lidocaine (Lidoderm), which when placed directly over the painful area, quickly numbs it out. The effect lasts for up to twelve hours and you can use as many as three patches at a time. Because the drug is applied only to the skin, it's not really absorbed into your body so it doesn't cause any drug interactions. A few patients get local reactions that make the skin red and irritated and the patches can't be used on an area of skin that's damaged in any way (often the case in people with late-phase neuropathy). We have to choose the patch areas carefully. Lidocaine patches are my go-to temporary solution for patients who have neuropathy pain that's localized enough that we can find the source (usually on the bottom of the foot) and cover it with a patch.

Some patients don't respond well to lidocaine patches. We can't know who will respond and who won't until we try. Fortunately, because this is a very safe treatment, we can just put on a patch and see what happens. If it works, great; the patient will usually get about twelve hours of pain relief. If it doesn't, we haven't done harm. A drawback to the patches is that they're very pricey, although insurance usually covers them.

Injections

My favorite technique for longer-term (but not permanent) pain relief is injecting a combination of *dexamethasone* and *xylocaine* into the painful area. Dexamethasone is a synthetic steroid that helps reduce swelling, which in turn decompresses the nerves. Xylocaine is the same thing as lidocaine, which numbs the area. We use ultrasound imaging to guide the injection and get the medicine right next to, but not into, the large nerve in the affected area. The shots don't really hurt and are very safe—reactions to either drug are rare. You may need several shots over a period of a few weeks to get the most relief, which can last from weeks to months.

Combined Electrochemical Treatment (CET)

Building on the injection concept, we now use a device that combines the benefits of a nerve block by using *bupivacaine* (a local anesthetic similar to lidocaine) with high-frequency electronic signal treatment (EST). Very high frequencies essentially "reboot" the nerve and this has an anti-inflammatory effect, relieving some of the swelling that causes compression. Over time, the technique also seems to lead to partial regeneration of small nerve fibers; with some patients, we also see improved conduction in the larger sensory nerves. This technique has been extremely effective for many of my patients. They usually have marked improvements in pain and quality of life. Sleep improves, and patients enjoy improved balance. They can once again walk, exercise, and easily do their everyday activities. Most important, it relieves pain long-term without the side effects of drugs.

Laser Therapy

When you have diabetic peripheral neuropathy, you have damage not just to the peripheral nerves in your feet, but also to the tiny blood vessels that nourish those nerves. When blood doesn't flow well to the damaged nerves, it's that much harder for your body to repair itself. In addition to bringing oxygen and nutrients to the nerves and carrying away waste products, your blood also brings in natural repair chemicals, such as insulin-like growth factor and nerve growth factor. If the microcirculation is impaired, so are these natural mechanisms. Improving the microcirculation to your feet helps relieve the pain of neuropathy and also to heal it.

The first step in restoring your microcirculation is improving your blood sugar numbers. When your blood is full of sugar, the tiny blood vessels everywhere in your body—your feet, eyes, kidneys, and heart—get plugged up with oxidized glucose. The next step is to take measures to help restore the circulation at a microscopic level.

There's no magic pill for this, but we do have an excellent new treatment that can be very helpful. My patients have had very good results with low-level laser therapy, also known as cold or soft laser therapy. The way this works is complex, but it basically comes down to the way blue light just below the visible spectrum can make the *hemoglobin* (the molecule that carries oxygen) in your red blood cells release nitric oxide. As we've discussed, when you have diabetes, your ability to produce nitric oxide is impaired by the excess sugar in your blood. Because nitric oxide is the natural chemical that relaxes the walls of your blood vessels, a deficiency will cause these vessels to constrict and restrict blood flow at the most basic cellular level. That's why organs with many very small blood vessels, like your eyes and kidneys, are so badly damaged by high blood sugar. But low levels of nitric oxide also damage your smallest nerves, such as the nerve fibers in your feet, by constricting blood circulation. Better circulation in your feet means less neuropathy pain and a better chance for your damaged nerves to regenerate.

By the time you reach phase 3, you have fibrous tissue in your feet caused by scarred and damaged nerves. The laser wavelengths can't easily penetrate this tissue, which reduces how well the treatment can work. For people in the early phases, laser therapy can be remarkably effective. The drawback is that it doesn't last very long.

Regenerative Medicine

For some of my patients, modern regenerative medicine—the cutting edge of medical science—can literally save their lives. Regenerative medicine means delivering specific types of cells or cell products to diseased tissues or organs. The aim is for the cells to restore themselves through the body's own healing processes.

Regenerative medicine has been around for decades. The first bone marrow transplant, for instance, took place more than forty years ago. More recently, stem cell research holds the promise of healing the body from within by helping it regenerate damaged cells, including nerve cells. Much of it is still experimental, but I now use two types of regenerative therapy for patients with diabetic ulcers that won't heal.

The first approach is a technique in which we inject platelet-rich plasma, or PRP, near the affected nerve. To accomplish this, we collect a small amount the patient's own blood (just a couple of vials) and use a centrifuge to concentrate the platelets and stem cells. Platelets, the tiny particles that help your blood clot, are rich in growth factors that are important for tissue repair.

For patients who are in very deep trouble with end-stage diabetic ulcers—facing amputation and possibly death—I use an advanced treatment called amniotic fluid therapy. The treatment material comes from amniotic fluid (the fluid that bathes a fetus in the womb) that is collected during cesarean sections, so it doesn't have any of the ethical issues associated with some other sources of stem cells. Amniotic fluid is very rich in pluripotent stem cells that can turn themselves into any sort of tissue in the body.

Other Helpful Alternatives

Capsaicin

Some of my patients try capsaicin cream as a way to relieve localized pain. Capsaicin is the ingredient that makes hot peppers hot, and when you rub the cream into the painful area, you can feel it giving off heat. This is mildly painful, which is actually the point. The stimulation caused by capsaicin depletes the nerves in the affected area of a neuro-chemical called *substance P*. Because substance P is involved with transmitting pain along a nerve, depleting it means that the nerve can't send the pain signal. The effect, if any, is only temporary.

Several studies have looked at capsaicin and some have found that it can be mildly helpful for neuropathy pain. However, in Minneapolis, researchers with the Mayo Clinic's Department of Neurology conducted the largest and best study in which they found that capsaicin wasn't any better than a placebo. It's available at any pharmacy without a prescription, so many of my patients try it. They don't report much success. If you want to try capsaicin, be very cautious. Follow the package directions. Be very sure you don't apply it to any area of the skin that is irritated or damaged in any way.

Neuro-Eze

As discussed in Chapter 2, your body needs plenty of the amino acid L-arginine to synthesize nitric oxide. One of the benefits of laser therapy is that it stimulates the release of nitric oxide—which in turn improves circulation. Yet there's a more direct way to get L-arginine to where it's needed in the small blood vessels of your feet. For my patients with phase 1 or phase 2 neuropathy, I often prescribe Neuro-Eze, a nonprescription product that's massaged directly onto the painful area on the foot. Available as a cream or liquid, Neuro-Eze releases an enzyme called *nitric oxide synthase*. When it's thoroughly rubbed in and absorbed into the bloodstream, the enzyme speeds up the process that converts L-arginine to nitric oxide. The effect starts almost at once and lasts for a couple of hours, and the Neuro-Eze needs to be applied two or three times a day. This is one of the most effective self-help measures for those with the early phases of small fiber neuropathy.

Acupuncture

The ancient art of painlessly inserting very thin needles at selected points just under the skin is sometimes recommended as a treatment for pain from peripheral neuropathy. In theory, acupuncture should work well, because it's believed that the needles stimulate the release of nitric oxide. In practice, some of my patients have had good experiences with this, with a definite reduction of pain, although no improvement in anything else, like numbness. Most of them, however, have had only marginal results or no results at all.

Most studies of acupuncture have considered it for treating neuropathy caused by chemotherapy, not diabetes. Those studies are very negative—it doesn't seem to help much if at all. The one major study that looked at acupuncture for diabetic peripheral neuropathy was published in 1998. Almost all the patients got some or even significant relief from the treatments. The problem is that the study was very small. Only 44 patients participated, which makes the results hard to interpret. In a group that small, some of the benefits could be due to medications they were taking, to the placebo effect, or even just to chance.

Why waste time and money on something that isn't likely to help?

Dietary Supplements

A few of my patients find dietary supplements to be helpful. The challenge is that some supplement manufacturers make exaggerated claims about how well their products work on peripheral neuropathy. Based on my experience, I can only recommend a handful of supplements that have enough science behind them to back up the hype.

1. **Prescription-level vitamin B.** A prescription supplement called Metanx, which contains a proprietary mix of the B vitamins folic acid (in the form of *L-methylfolate*) along with B$_6$ (*pyroxidine*) and B$_{12}$ (*cobalamin*), can sometimes help people with phase 1 or phase 2 neuropathy. The B vitamins are crucial for proper nerve function, but some of them—the ones in Metanx—are hard for your body

to absorb from food. This ability to absorb decreases if you have type 2 diabetes, but it also naturally declines with age,* which is why I often prescribe Metanx or any similar prescription B vitamins. One exception is *cobalamin* (B_{12}), which is found only in animal foods—so some vegetarians and all vegans need to supplement to be sure they're getting enough.†

2. **Over-the-counter vitamin B.** Instead, I recommend a high-quality B-100 supplement, which you can buy at any pharmacy or health food store. These supplements contain 100 percent of the daily recommended amount of all the B vitamins. A good brand is Rodex Forte. We don't have much evidence for B vitamins helping diabetic peripheral neuropathy. However, I've seen that some patients really do benefit from taking them. It could be that these patients are running low on B vitamins, but aren't yet deficient; so the supplement raises their levels back up to normal.

3. **Alpha-lipoic acid (ALA)** is a very close cousin of the B vitamins. It's not officially a vitamin because you can manufacture tiny amounts of it in your body instead of getting it from food; but in fact, most of the lipoic acid in your body comes from what you eat. Alpha-lipoic

---

*In foods such as dark green leafy vegetables, folic acid is found in the form of folate. Some people are genetically slow converters of folate to folic acid, so they may run on the low side for this nutrient.

†Once you hit middle age, your production of intrinsic factor, a substance produced in your stomach that's needed to absorb cobalamin from your food, gradually slows down and can even stop. Some of the symptoms of cobalamin deficiency resemble peripheral neuropathy—and they can slowly develop even if a blood test for cobalamin says you have normal levels.

acid is found in small amounts in many foods, including broccoli, Brussels sprouts, carrots, tomatoes, and spinach. It's also found in red meat.

In your body, ALA has two roles: it's needed to recycle *glutathione*, your body's most abundant antioxidant, and to keep your *mitochondria* (tiny power plants producing energy in your cells) working efficiently. While alpha-lipoic acid is on its own a very powerful antioxidant, most of your ALA is busy recycling glutathione and making your mitochondria work right—so there's not much left over for that role. This is where the supplements shine. Remember our discussion in Chapter 2 about how the polyol pathway leads to the formation of AGEs and glycation? Because ALA is fat soluble, it's good at getting through the fatty myelin sheath protecting your large nerves and into the nerve cells, where it can help prevent AGEs damage. However, to have enough extra ALA in your system for this to occur, you might need to take supplements.

4. **Fish oil.** Some of my patients find that taking fish oil supplements seems to help their neuropathy. Frankly, no long-term study has been done yet. Fish oil has other benefits, such as lowering triglycerides, but so far, helping peripheral neuropathy symptoms isn't among them. A key substance in fatty fish (as well as walnuts and flaxseed oil) is omega-3, which along with omega-6, is called an essential fatty acid. Much more in Chapter 9 and the discussion of diet.

5. **Evening primrose oil.** This supplement, high in omega-6 fatty acids, is sometimes recommended as a natural treatment for peripheral neuropathy. However, the primary

study claiming it helps relieve symptoms involved only 111 participants and was published in 1993; still, this might be worth trying.*

6. **Magnesium.** People with diabetes are usually low in the important mineral magnesium—by some estimates, this number is as high as 80 percent.† If you already have neuropathy, being low on magnesium can make it worse. Among my patients, almost everyone who has foot ulcers is also magnesium deficient. Taking a magnesium supplement is one way to raise your level, and so I recommend 1,000 mg a day of magnesium citrate, a form of magnesium that's easy on your digestive system.‡

    If you have high blood pressure, taking magnesium supplements may bring it down somewhat. Cutting sugar from your diet may also bring your blood pressure down, so keep an eye on it. If you start to feel dizzy or lightheaded, it's possible your blood pressure has dropped too low, so consult your physician should that occur.

---

*The anti-inflammatory effect of the omega-6 amino acid, *gamma Linolenic acid* (GLA), seems to be what helps. The dose in the study was 480 milligrams a day.

†The number is not all that different from people *without* diabetes. Most Americans take in less magnesium than the recommended dietary allowance (420 mg for an adult man and 320 for an adult woman). This is a direct result of the large amounts of refined carbohydrates we eat—almost all the magnesium found in whole grains is processed away.

‡Too much magnesium can cause an upset stomach or diarrhea, so begin with a lower dose to see how you react.

When Is It Time for Surgery?

The time for having the Dellon Decompression Surgical Procedure is when your neuropathy has reached the point of severely limiting your mobility or if you have multiple ulcerations on your legs or feet.

When your nerves are so compressed that your feet and toes are mostly numb, you can't feel the floor when you walk. Like the cowboy in Chapter 6, this affects your balance and puts you at risk of having a nasty fall (if you haven't had one already). On several occasions I've needed to delay surgery until a patient's fall-related broken hip, fractured wrist, or concussion healed. Furthermore, when your feet are numb, you can't feel the pedals in your car. You can no longer drive.

Even if your feet aren't numb, if they're painful enough to keep you up at night it's time to consider decompression surgery. And if cutaneous pressure-threshold testing shows that the large sensory nerves in your feet are seriously deteriorating, surgery can keep them from getting worse and may well restore sensation and relieve the pain.* If possible, the surgery should be done while you still have a positive *Tinel's sign*† validating that the nerve is still functioning. That way, we know there's an 80 percent chance of success.

However, I have had a few patients in such dire condition that the nerve was too damaged for them to feel anything

---

*Remember, if you have numbness, you have large fiber involvement, even if you have abnormal small fibers (related to pain, not numbness). If you have numbness and pain, you have a mixed fiber neuropathy.

†Named for the French neurologist Jules Tinel, this is the "little hammer test" in which your doctor lightly taps over a nerve to evoke a tingling sensation.

when I pressed on it—they had no Tinel's sign at all. The only alternative to the Dellon procedure was amputation. Those patients agreed to go ahead with the Dellon procedure even though I couldn't be sure it would help at all. To my surprise, in addition to a relief of pain, every patient regained some sensation! They probably didn't gain as much as they would have if we had operated sooner, but the more important point is that their ulcerated feet began to heal and stayed healed. Amputation was avoided.

You Need Not Suffer

When I was a young man learning to be a foot surgeon, I was taught that peripheral neuropathy was an almost inevitable consequence of long-term diabetes. It couldn't be prevented, nor could it be treated effectively. People with diabetic peripheral neuropathy would only get worse. My job would be to treat these patients as they developed worsening symptoms. Eventually, when all other treatments failed, my job as a surgeon would be to amputate their toes and feet.

And as I began my practice, everything I'd been taught about neuropathy seemed to be true. My patients with diabetic neuropathy did almost always get slowly worse. Their pain and numbness increased over time. Some would get foot ulcers that took weeks or even months to heal; some would need amputations.

And as their feet got worse, my patients felt guilty and helpless. Try as they might to take their meds and eat the way they were told, they still were in pain. They couldn't work and they couldn't drive. They lost mobility and independence as they came to depend on walkers and wheelchairs. They ended up in the hospital with infected foot ulcerations that led to amputations and sometimes even death. I felt guilt as well as helplessness.

Over the years, I also noticed that some of my patients had, against all medical advice, started following a low-carb/paleo diet. They lost weight, got their blood sugar under control, and saw their neuropathy improve. Despite dire warnings, their kidneys didn't fail, their bones stayed strong, and they didn't get colon cancer.

Eliminating sugar from your diet is not only a tangible step, it's also the single most effective treatment I can recommend for peripheral neuropathy. I don't have to write you a prescription, give you an injection, shine a laser on your foot, or perform surgery. All I have to do is explain what causes global compression and encourage you to cut the sugar. After that, it's entirely in your hands. The responsibility for your own health is now something you can actively manage for yourself. You can take simple, achievable steps to end your reliance on brain-altering drugs and repeated visits to my office.

I love nothing more than losing patients to better health.

PART III

So Now What's Stopping You?

8

The Sugar Addiction

#KICKINGTHEHABIT

Okay. You're convinced. You always knew too much sugar was bad, but now you understand how and why. And yet the thought of cutting sugar from your diet has you longing for a Twinkie or *pastel des tres leches*. That's because sugar is addictive. And so—as with any other drug—the first step toward gaining control is recognizing that sugar—like any other drug—has taken hold of your behavior as well as your physiology. You grab Cheetos when things get tense. You can't lose a quick five pounds anymore. You see the signs of damage.

Why Are You Addicted to Sugar?

Sweet foods taste good, of course, but what really causes addiction is the way sugar makes you feel. If you're tired and hungry, chocolate or ice cream gives an energy boost. The "sweet monkey on your back" comes from deep within your hard wiring. Mother's milk, the first taste we encounter, is sweet—and in fact, researchers have discovered that when newborns are given a sugar solution immediately before a painful experience (such as a diagnostic heel prick) they cry less. As a child, you were probably rewarded or comforted with candy or cookies. Being a good boy at the dentist. Sitting still when Grandmother came to dinner. As an adult, you may still find comfort in sweets when you're upset, sad, lonesome, or feeling neglected or unloved.

On top of that, sugary foods are almost impossible to avoid. In the supermarket, shelf after shelf and aisle after aisle, we see nothing but sugar in various forms: candy, cookies, snack foods, soft drinks, juices, breakfast cereals, energy bars, sweetened yogurt. And that's not even counting the hidden sugar in savory and prepared foods. Even the produce section of the supermarket has been infiltrated by sugar. Salad dressings with added sugar are placed temptingly close to the lettuce; kits for making candy apples are perched next to the fruit itself. In the workplace, sweet foods are everywhere. At staff meetings, doughnuts and bagels are likely to be on the side table next to the coffee; the leftovers end up in the break room next to the brownies brought in by well-meaning coworkers. The receptionist has a candy dish on her desk. And how can you refuse a piece of cake at an office birthday party?

You know sugar's bad for you and you want to give it up, but you can't. In fact, sometimes you end up eating a lot more of it than you planned or even really wanted. When you don't get your sugar fix, you feel shaky and physically ill. You're also anxious and irritable—driven to find something sweet, you eat it at once. Can you concentrate on work knowing there's a chocolate bar in your desk drawer? Probably not—and the only solution is to eat it.

Hunger vs. Craving

So many diets focus on willpower. And if you fail, it's because you really just *didn't want to succeed*. We used to call that being *judgmental*. Yes, you must want to change—but when body chemistry is involved, that may not be enough.

Let's take a minute to examine the idea of what it means to be satiated or full. This process is governed in part by *leptin*, a hormone produced by your body fat. It signals your brain that you have plenty of stored fat and don't need to eat any more. Leptin turns off your hunger switch and signals the stomach to stop growling because you're satiated. However, consuming too much fructose causes a fatty liver, which in turn leads to leptin resistance. Similar to what happens in insulin resistance, your body produces more and more leptin, but your brain doesn't get the message, according to Robert Lustig, M.D., a member of the Endocrine Society's Obesity Task Force. Insulin resistance generates leptin resistance, meaning the more sugar you eat, the hungrier you feel—truly a vicious cycle.*

What happens in your body to cause this? Sugar stimulates your brain to release the body's natural "feel-good chemicals": dopamine, serotonin, and endorphins,† which in turn make you want to eat more sugar so that you produce more of the chemicals. When you eat sugary foods, you're consuming a white powder that's every bit as addictive as cocaine. Serotonin and endorphins, in particular, are two of the

---

*In the next chapter we'll look at a second hormone, *cholecystokinin* (CCK), which aids in the digestion of animal fat and protein—with completely different results.

†There is a fourth "feel-good hormone," *oxytocin*, which is released during sexual orgasm.

six primary neurotransmitters (molecules carrying signals across nerve junctions or synapse) and they are responsible for modulating mood and brain chemistry.* It's exactly the same pathway activated by opiates, such as cocaine, heroin, and morphine. It's also the same pathway activated by nicotine from tobacco products. If you've ever tried to quit smoking, you know how difficult it is to overcome your body's desire for its addictive chemicals. Sugar is perfectly legal—you can't get arrested for driving with a sugar rush—but it's just as addictive as the others. The damage to your body comes in the form of obesity, diabetes, and crushed nerves.

Researchers at the University of Bordeaux, in France, found that even lab rats addicted to cocaine will choose saccharine-infused† water over the drug.

Clearly, sugar isn't something you can give up easily, but if you have diabetic neuropathy, you have no choice. Sugar is crushing your nerves and putting you on the downhill path to constant pain, disability, diabetic foot ulcers, amputation, and death. I think that's a pretty good motivation for giving up the sweet stuff.

Craving is an even more complex process. For example, a high-carb diet can make you feel physically full, but not really *satisfied*. The important point is to be aware that you're going to feel different during the first couple of weeks of eliminating sugar. Not only will you crave sugar, but you will also crave that "full feeling."

We have all been raised to be habitually dependent on

---

*Many researchers, including those at the University of Wales, record that poor mood stimulates desire for high-carbohydrate/high-fat foods, thus triggering production of both.

†Saccharine is 300 times sweeter than sucrose.

sugar and breaking such dependency can be a challenge. As you cut sugar and add good animal fats, your body will begin to adjust. You'll stop experiencing surges and plummets in your energy level; your thinking will seem sharper; you'll begin losing weight; and most important, you'll be reducing the inflammation that is a chief factor in global compression.

The Social Impact of Changing Sugar Patterns

Of course, eating is more than just a way to fuel your body. Eating is also a social activity and a form of entertainment. Just look at the hundreds of cookbooks, cooking shows, and restaurants that we love to read, watch, and visit. We bond with friends and family over meals and we feel a form of social obligation as well as comfort when we eat with others. "Breaking bread" is the time-honored term for conflict resolution.

Rest assured that as you become more aware of the sugar you're consuming and the negative impacts on your health, you'll still have meals to bond over and flavor adventures to enjoy, with the added benefit of many more years of healthy life to enjoy them.

The key to kicking sugar is replacing it with better choices. Some foods can simply be switched with organic versions, such as tomato sauce with no added sugar. Sugary baked goods and snacks must simply be cut out of your life. Giving up other foods is difficult, especially if they're associated with specific times and activities. If after dinner you regularly have a big bowl of ice cream while relaxing in front of the TV, you'll find yourself craving ice cream the minute you settle down on the couch. One way to kill the craving is to shake up your routine. Instead of watching TV, do something else, such as going for a walk or calling a friend. Or if you really want to watch TV in your usual way, swap the ice cream for something healthier with less sugar.

As you cut back on sugar, make sure you don't get too hungry. That's a sure way to start feeling a blood sugar crash that can only be fixed with something sweet. When you're at work or away from home, take some protein with you. Otherwise, a snack attack could send you foraging through vending machines full of junk because there's nothing else available.

Avoid sugary situations. Okay, this can't happen all the time, but do you really need to walk past the cupcake shop every day? Cross the street or take a different route. Sugary foods are offered to you all the time, but if you can avoid them easily, try to do so. At a birthday party, you can't avoid the cake, but spend your energy handing it out to others. A simple step like that can help you stick to a single small piece. If you're meeting a friend for coffee, try to avoid doing it in a bakery café full of temptation. Maybe you could meet in the park instead?

How to Cope with Cravings

Addicts crave what they're addicted to, so you should expect sugar cravings as you work on eliminating it from your life. Experts disagree about how to define addiction, but one thing they do agree on is that stopping the substance leads to withdrawal symptoms. While you may feel tired, irritable, depressed, headachy, and anxious at times as you cut sugar from your diet, you can get through a few days of feeling crummy, especially if you know that you are doing something positive for your health.

There's no instant cure for these feelings, although as time goes by they will almost certainly fade away. It doesn't usually take long—within a week you'll probably be feeling them a lot less. In the meantime, here are a few ideas that have worked for my patients:

- If you have diabetes, check your blood sugar if you get a craving. You could be on the low side. If so, take your usual steps to bring up your blood sugar. Be aware, however, that kicking the sugar habit too abruptly could make your blood sugar drop too low (hypoglycemia). This is not a good thing, so use your glucose meter to keep an eye on how you're doing and avoid hypoglycemia. If you do drop too low, it's okay to eat a small amount of something sweet to bring your blood sugar back up.

  Once you're back to normal, the craving will subside. If you get frequent episodes of low blood sugar, discuss with your diabetes specialist ways to avoid them. Sugar cravings aside, hypoglycemia is bad for your body in many other ways.

- Have a high-protein breakfast to keep the cravings away. Eggs are an effective and healthy choice (even the American Heart Association says so). But why not try some baked chicken legs, or a protein shake with frozen blueberries, or organic peanut butter on apple slices? Have it with some hot buttered coffee (our star of Chapter 10), which will stave off sugar cravings for hours. If you do get a sugar craving, eating something with protein can help.

- Eat good fats. A sugar craving is sometimes your body's way of asking for the fat it hasn't been getting. Instead of a cookie, have some avocado, or some full-fat goat cheese, or a green salad with lots of olive oil and a dash of vinegar.

A hard-boiled egg is also a good option. Fats are very sati-
ating, so you'll squash the craving and your appetite at the
same time.

- Eat regularly to avoid hunger pangs that scream to be fixed
quickly with a candy bar or doughnut. Plan ahead so that
sugarless meals and snacks are fast and easy.

- Stay hydrated. Sometimes when you think you're hungry
and want a candy bar, it's because you're actually thirsty.
Especially while you're kicking sugar, drink plenty of plain
water, coffee, tea, or herbal tea—anything without sugar or
artificial sweeteners.

- Are you really hungry for something sweet? Maybe you're
just tired, irritated, bored, lonesome, or sad—these are the
emotional triggers that send you to sugary foods. Sometimes all you really need is a nap instead of a cupcake; just
be aware of how the way you feel affects what you eat.
Simply realizing that you're eating for emotional reasons,
rather than true hunger, can be enough to short-circuit a
sugar craving.

- Add a pinch of salt. Surprisingly, a small amount of salt
brings out the natural sweetness of some foods, especially
fruit. If your fruit smoothie seems too tart, add a bit of salt
and taste it again—it will be sweeter.

- Brush your teeth. I have a patient who found this really
helped. I've told other patients about it and they swear it
works.

- Try taking supplements of the amino acid L-glutamine
(this isn't the same thing at all as MSG). Glutamine is an
essential part of the complex process that tells your body
your blood sugar has dropped and you need to bring it
back up to normal by releasing more glycogen, the form of

glucose stored in your liver. Releasing glycogen stabilizes your blood sugar and helps cut the cravings.

- Get enough sleep. Studies have shown that you find it much harder to resist sweet and salty snacks when you're tired or sleep deprived. So if you're well rested, you'll be better able to fend off carb cravings. One notable study conducted at the University of California, Berkeley's Sleep and Neuro-imaging Laboratory used MRI scans to measure the brain activity levels of sleep-deprived participants as they were shown images of healthy and unhealthy foods, then asked to rank the foods according to desirability. Subjects exhibited *impaired* activity in the brain's frontal lobe (which governs complex decision making) along with *increased* activity in those brain regions responding to rewards. In short, they *physically* craved junk food. And German researchers found that both shortened and disturbed night sleep compromises your ability to metabolize glucose.*

- It's okay to give in once in a while. If a craving is severe or disruptive, have something sweet or decadent—but make it count. Have a square of high-quality dark chocolate or a small scoop of premium ice cream (the kind with a lot of butterfat), an amuse-bouche, or a glass of wine. Then let it go. Try another strategy next time.

And last but not least:

- Avoid artificial sweeteners.

---

*Pity the poor volunteers in the German study who simply were awakened every two hours to have their blood glucose levels tested. At least the Berkeley subjects were rewarded with their personal junk food choices after their MRI scans.

As you try to cut back on sugar, you may be tempted to switch to products made with artificial, no-calorie sweeteners. Don't. Swapping sugar for artificial sweeteners such as saccharin, acesulfame (Sunett), aspartame (NutraSweet, Equal, Neotame), or sucralose (Splenda and Apriva) could actually lead to *more* weight gain and inflammation. The same is true for stevia, an herbal product that is much sweeter than sugar.

Artificial sweeteners are bad for many reasons, including:

1. They can alter your metabolism. A groundbreaking study conducted on both mice and humans by researchers at Israel's Weizmann Institute of Science concluded that artificial sweeteners can alter the composition of your "gut microbiota," hastening the development of glucose intolerance—and thus may contribute significantly to obesity and diabetes. The scientists called for a "public reassessment of the massive and unsupervised use of artificial sweeteners."

2. They can alter brain activity. Sparked by a 1992 U.S. Air Force–issued publication, "Aspartame Alert," pilots throughout the world have been warned to avoid artificial sweeteners of all kinds because they can induce among other things, flicker vertigo, memory loss, and dizziness while flying.

3. They perpetuate your addictive taste for sweetness.

In the Multi-Ethnic Study of Atherosclerosis (MESA), from 2009, participants who drank diet drinks every day had a 36 percent higher risk for metabolic syndrome and a 67 percent greater risk for type 2 diabetes. Other studies have shown similar results.*

Why do artificial sweeteners cause blood sugar problems? Possibly because their supersweet taste stimulates your body to prepare for calories that never arrive. This disrupts all of the hormonal and neurological signals that tell you you're full. The drink doesn't fill you up—in fact, it make you feel hungrier, so you eat more, which adds more calories. Also, many people associate drinking soft drinks with eating high-calorie and highly processed food, such as pizza or fast food. Having a diet soda at a fast-food restaurant won't make up for the extra-large serving of French fries. And because the diet drink doesn't suppress your appetite by providing calories, you're more likely to gulp down every one of those fries. And then order a cookie or milk shake to go.

It's also possible that artificial sweeteners can make your neuropathy worse as there has been some evidence that aspartame and other fake sweeteners are neurotoxins that can damage nerves or even kill them off. In my own clinical observations, I've noticed that my neuropathy patients who do nothing but switch from artificially sweetened drinks to plain water tend to improve.

Let's Get Down to Business

Express Route

For me, cold turkey was the most satisfying approach. I decided to stop and I just did it. So that's my first advice to all

*Of course, a 2014 study sponsored by the American Beverage Association said that diet soda can *help* weight loss. An industry-sponsored study that just happens to come to the conclusion the industry wants? Can you seriously think this study, which got a lot of publicity, is anything but propaganda?

patients. You'll gain strength every day as your body adjusts to its new chemistry. You'll learn how to say no to the social conventions—without guilt.

Is kicking sugar easy? Definitely not—but it can and must be done. For many of my patients, the hardest part is just recognizing how much sugar they really eat each day. They're horrified when they realize how they have unknowingly damaged their nerves. Once past that, they're ready to move on to concrete steps to conquer sugar addiction.

After a couple of weeks of eating no sugar, you'll make the surprising discovery that you've become much more sensitive to the taste. Cookies now taste overly sweet, and you realize that many other processed foods in your diet, such as tomato sauce and even cream of mushroom soup, contain *added* sugar. Your taste buds become more sensitive to other flavors as well when not overloaded by sugar. Food in general will probably taste better and you'll find yourself enjoying a wider variety of culinary treats.

Phasing in Change

The express train worked for me, but if that's not you, a gradual approach is also fine. Reduce your sugar intake slowly but steadily. Taper off the amount of sugar you put in your coffee and pass on dessert every other day until you're passing on it every day. Give away the last of the Halloween candy, or better yet—don't buy it at all next year. Give the trick-or-treaters healthy snacks, comics, or small games and puzzles.

I'm fortunate enough to have the assistance of Judy Nicassio, a nutritionist, who comes to my office and counsels patients who must transition from their day-to-day decisions and opt for dietary change—meaning eliminating sugar from their diets. Judy's nutrition plans will be detailed in Chapter 10, but regarding controlling sugar addiction she advises patients to:

- concentrate on smaller portion sizes;
- make a list of the order in which you cut out sugary foods: candy the first week, ice cream the second, and so on;
- recognize that all carbohydrates convert to sugar and are addictive;
- avoid white food: white flour, white sugar, white potatoes, white rice, and white pasta.

One Step at a Time

One of my patients was a famous actor and she told me an interesting story about Lucille Ball that relates to breaking the sugar habit. After becoming a comedic icon, Lucy taught master acting classes for many years and she implored her students to learn the art of purposeful selfishness—to ask themselves with every decision, "How does this help me."

Many of my patients spend a lifetime helping others, and you may be the same. It's now time to help you. Motivation to change your diet must come from within. This time, think about what's good for *your* health and well-being.

When you decide to eliminate sugar from your normal diet, you can still enjoy social events and cooking for family and friends, but don't be afraid to politely refuse a piece of pie if you need to. Bake the holiday gifts, just don't eat half of them yourself.

There are many formalized step programs for overcoming any kind of addiction; but one of my favorites is from Helpguide.org, an education center founded by Jeanne Segal and Robert Segal, after the death of their daughter, Morgan.

1. Always remember *why* you want to quit.
2. If you've tried quitting before, focus on what *worked* that time.
3. Establish simple, measurable goals—such as dates for the phases of recovery.
4. Rid your home and workplace of all reminders of your addiction.

9

The Big Fat Lie

EDUCATED INTO IGNORANCE

To understand why a diet that's high in carbohydrates and low in saturated fat is so misdirected, we need to discuss how we got here as a society. And we need to appreciate how all of us have been manipulated by forces you may have never considered.

Lie #1: Animal Fat Is Bad

It's easy to visualize animal fat clogging your arteries like bacon fat clogging a kitchen sink drain, but the science doesn't work that way. And yet, based on what I hear from my patients, there's more misinformation out there about fat than just about any other aspect of your health. Let's clear up the fat myth once and for all.

Fat doesn't make you fat; carbohydrates make you fat.

The Unproven Hypothesis

We should begin with a brief review of the scientific method, something you studied in middle school science class. Since the seventeenth century, we've validated scientific inquiry by presenting a hypothesis—something concluded from clinical observation—and then inviting the community to challenge (in other words, test) the idea to prove its validity. So a hypothesis is an exploration of a phenomenon and the scientific method involving review by peers proves it—or not. The whole point of the *method* is to inspire and nourish new thinking, which is then substantiated.

For the past several decades you've probably been making food choices based on a well-touted and fully declared "truth" that's been sanctioned by lawmakers, scientific experts, industrial agriculture, and the marketplace. A sanction seized upon by food producers that's led us to a world of low-fat, processed foods—and inevitably to obesity and diabetes.

Based upon the Aristotelian principle of the syllogism, the "saturated fat-heart hypothesis" goes like this:

1. Saturated animal fat in the diet increases cholesterol in the blood.*

---

*Saturated fats are saturated with hydrogen molecules and naturally present themselves as solid at room temperature. Unsaturated fats lack some of these hydrogens, are liquid at room temperatures, and are known commonly as oils. *Trans fats*, the evil spawn, occur rarely in nature (in milk and some meat products) but in our industrialized world is the contaminant produced in "hydrogenation"—the adding of hydrogen to make oil solid so it can ship easier, last longer on the grocery shelf, and have a better "mouth feel" (crunchier or creamier, as the case may be). But your government allows trans fats to be marketed as natural or "partially hydrogenated oils," when in fact they are natural oil (like corn oil) turned into something unnatural. Dare I say unholy?

2. High cholesterol increases your risk of having a heart attack.

3. Therefore, saturated fat in the diet increases your risk of having a heart attack.

Although many well-meaning physicians, nutritionists, and modern grandmothers believe this logical sequence is the gospel truth, there is no scientific proof of the original observation. It is a false analogy. No study has *proved* that saturated fat increases cholesterol and in turn causes heart disease. Overall, the primary argument simply fails scrutiny under the scientific method.

Take the first statement, that eating saturated fat from animal foods raises blood cholesterol. Study after study has looked for this vital link, and study after study has failed to find it. I don't believe the relationship exits.

The discussion prompting reexamination of the long-term association of saturated (primarily animal) fat with cardiovascular disease began in 2010 with the publication of a statistical meta-analysis of 21 studies involving almost 350,000 test subjects. The researchers, led by Patty Siri-Tarino of Children's Hospital Oakland Research Institute, stated, "There is no significant evidence for concluding that dietary saturated fat is associated with an increased risk of CHD [coronary heart disease] or CVD [cardiovascular disease]."

What I find interesting is that the report goes on to conclude that more study is needed to see if cardiovascular disease has been influenced by the specific foods people eat instead of animal protein. Often I tell patients, "If it tastes too good, don't eat it." And I'm not really joking. Far too many of the processed foods we eat have been deliberately manipulated by the food industry to be *hyperpalatable,* or at the "Bliss Point."* That means they've been designed to provide exactly the right combination of salt, sugar, and fat that makes the food irresistibly delicious. And when the country began the bogus "fat-free" phase, fat was replaced with, you guessed it—more sugar. These foods don't just taste good; they taste *great* because they've been carefully designed to make you addicted. And because of addiction, you eat as much as you possibly can.

A recent analysis conducted by researchers in the United Kingdom, United States, and the Netherlands that included 76 past studies with almost 650,000 participants concluded, "Current evidence does not clearly support cardiovascular guidelines that encourage high consumption of polyunsaturated fatty acids and low consumption of total saturated fats."

Now take the second statement of the saturated fat–heart syllogism—that high cholesterol increases your risk of having a heart attack. It's true in some cases, and yet well over half of all people having a first heart attack have *normal* cholesterol levels. And as many people with high cholesterol never have a heart attack.

When high cholesterol is combined with other factors, your heart attack risk does jump statistically. In particular, high cholesterol raises your risk of heart disease if you're also overweight; have diabetes or the metabolic syndrome; eat a diet full of low-quality carbohydrates leading to high triglycerides, insulin resistance, and high blood sugar; are

---

*Attributed to the market researcher and psychophysicist Howard Moskowitz, after his detailed study of the flavors in spaghetti sauces, the Bliss Point is that quantity of consumption after which any more will make the consumer feel *less* satisfied.

sedentary; have high blood pressure; and are exposed to environmental toxins such as cigarette smoke and alcohol.

What *Is* Cholesterol, Anyway?

Cholesterol is a waxy substance manufactured by your body. It's *not* a fat and it has no calories—your body doesn't burn cholesterol for energy. Instead, it uses cholesterol for a wide range of vital functions, including making your cell membranes and the fatty sheaths (myelin) that wrap around your nerves; manufacturing the hormones aldosterone, cortisol, testosterone, estrogen, and progesterone; and producing vitamin D. Cholesterol also produces the bile acids you need for digesting your food and it releases the neurotransmitters that send messages back and forth along your nerves. You can't live without cholesterol.

Contrary to the propaganda about eating low-cholesterol foods, almost all the cholesterol in your body is manufactured in your liver, and this can amount to between 800 to 1,500 mg per day. Most people take in another 300 to 450 mg or more from the animal foods they eat,* but only about half of that (or even less) is actually absorbed by your body. If you eat a substantial amount of high-cholesterol foods, your body compensates by making less cholesterol.

In order to transport waxy cholesterol through your watery bloodstream, your liver wraps it up in protein to create *lipoproteins*, of which there are two basic forms:

1. low-density lipoprotein, or LDL cholesterol, and
2. high-density lipoprotein, or HDL cholesterol.

*Plants, by definition, don't contain cholesterol.

A third and important factor associated with your cholesterol count are *triglycerides*, tiny fat particles in the blood that store energy and transport it to your muscles. High levels of triglycerides associated with high LDL are linked to heart disease and diabetes. Researchers believe triglycerides can elevate dangerously when you consume sugar, grains, and excessive alcohol; become sedentary; smoke; or become obese.

How Did Cholesterol Become a Culprit?

You'll often see LDL cholesterol referred to as the *bad* cholesterol and HDL cholesterol referred to as the *good* cholesterol. That's because LDL cholesterol moves fat from your liver to your cells, where it is taken up as needed—while HDL cholesterol carries the unused fat back to your liver, where about half of it gets recycled to make more LDL cholesterol. Some is then used to make bile acids while some gets recycled for other uses.

When you have high levels of LDL cholesterol, particularly if they are small, dense particles, you're at increased risk of heart disease—but not from the cholesterol itself. High cholesterol is just a big flashing sign telling you that you're in trouble from other risk factors. In fact, treating people with drugs to lower their cholesterol and prevent heart attacks is a flawed, long-running Big Pharma business plan.

How Does Cholesterol Relate to Cardiovascular Disease?

First it is important to note that cardiovascular disease (blockage of the arteries and heart) refers to disease that affects the lining of the blood vessels. This disease is not caused by fat, but rather by sugar. And the message we've been fed about the culpability of cholesterol is generally false. "Managing Your Cholesterol," a special health report recently released by Harvard Medical School, concludes that among other things, your doctor "may not be as concerned about your cholesterol 'numbers' as he or she once was." Instead, "elevated blood sugar can damage the lining of your arteries and make your blood more likely to clot."

What causes cardiovascular disease is the sugar and high-fructose corn syrup in your diet. As discussed in Chapter 2, this creates inflammatory reactions that damage the endothelium (the inner lining of your blood vessels). Your body's attempts to repair such damage end up backfiring and causing plaque—accumulations of cholesterol, white blood cells, and other gunk that get caught by the damaged, sticky endothelium. This is what can block an artery, and if the artery gets completely blocked, or if the plaque ruptures and causes a blood clot, blood flow is cut off. As a result, you can have a heart attack if the artery is one that nourishes your heart—or a stroke if it's one that nourishes your brain.

When you have coronary bypass surgery to reroute the blood supply to your heart, or when you have a stent inserted into a blocked artery to prop it open, you're still not solving the underlying problem of inflammation caused by too much sugar in your diet. You're just mechanically fixing one problem area—another is very likely to arise.

Just remember this—cholesterol is an essential substance and your cholesterol levels have nothing to do with the cholesterol in your diet. Yet in 2013 drug companies took in $23 billion from the sale of statin drugs. Stop and think about that for a minute. Or as the saying goes, follow the money.

If you want to have a lean body without the compressed arteries, nerves, and veins that lead to cardiovascular disease and stroke, you must rethink what you've been "mistaught" about fats. Stop eating carbs and start eating high-quality, grass-fed animal fat.* I know you've spent a lifetime fearing fats, but we've all been sold a lie and it's time we woke up and changed course.

What Are Omega-6 and Omega-3 Fatty Acids and Why Do They Matter?

Both omega-6 and omega-3 fatty acids are essential nutrients—you have to have both and the only way to get them is through food. Overall, omega-6s are needed for the inflammatory response, while omega-3s are needed for anti-inflammatory responses in the body.†

Boyd Eaton was author of a 1985 article on Paleolithic nutrition for *The New England Journal of Medicine* and in 1988 he coauthored the popular book *The Paleolithic Prescription*. Eaton conducted the original research showing that back in the Paleolithic era, before we domesticated animals or cultivated vegetables and grains, omega-6 and omega-3 fatty acids were at a 1:1 ratio in the human diet.

Today, because of our high intake of the cheap vegetable oils used in processed foods (which are high in omega-6s), the

---

*There is much more about what I mean by grass-fed in Chapter 10.

†This could be a separate book, but basically, the inflammatory response is your body's fundamental reaction for fighting off foreign particles, including disease. Anti-inflammatory refers to the reduction of inflammation or swelling. When your system become overwhelmed, pharmaceuticals (primarily analgesics) come to the rescue. These are essential tenets of modern medicine and many of us would die without such drugs.

ratio is radically lopsided and thus unnecessarily inflammatory. Many people with diabetes have an omega-6 ratio that is far too high—ranging anywhere from a 15:1 to 20:1 ratio to omega-3s. How and why does that make a difference?

The omega-6s and omega-3s are both mediated by the *delta-6 desaturase enzyme*. This enzyme, called delta for short, is like the bouncer at the door of a big party. He has to let both the omega-3s and the omega-6s into our bodies. Again, omega-3s are anti-inflammatory, like calm, well-behaved young men. The omega-6s are inflammatory, like rambunctious, party-hardy bikers. As long as an equal number of omega-3s and omega-6s are at the party, things stay under control. However, as more and more omega-6s arrive, they overwhelm the bouncer and disrupt the party. They crowd out the calm omega-3s and wreak havoc on the house (your body), including the plumbing system (urinary tract, with irritable bowel problems), the heating system (your autonomic nervous system), and the central computer system (your brain).

To prevent and ward off early inflammation (to be prophylactic), many doctors and nutritionists advocate anti-inflammatory diets high in omega-3s, including the Zone diet, developed by Barry Sears, M.D., and the work of Andrew Weil, M.D. My own anti-inflammatory diet will be the subject of Chapter 10.

Fat and Satiation

Saturated fat also plays a significant role in how your hormones tell your brain that you're full and don't need to eat again. In the last chapter we discussed the hormone leptin—and *cholecystokin* (CCK). They are both hormonal regula-

— chimps — 99% of our DNA

ONLY EAT MEAT

MEAT

9 × A YEAR

tors, released by your small intestine to ~~trigger~~ satiation.*
Researchers at University Hospital, Basel, Switzerland, concluded in an article published in the journal of *Physiology &
Behavior* that CCK is particularly effective in high-fat diets.
This process does involve a delay between eating and feeling
full, and so it's not surprising that many nutritionists advise
taking time to eat slowly and savor your food.

A diet high in animal fat *doesn't* make you feel full, but it
does make you feel satisfied—for longer. I experienced this
personally when I changed my own diet, and most of my patients who remove sugar from their diets and substitute saturated fats concur that they also remain satiated longer. A diet
high in sugar keeps you in a constant state of hunger. The
goal of the high-fat diet presented in Chapter 10 is to bring
you to the state of true satiation. It will transform your life.
You don't have to fast or starve—just put grass-fed animal fat
in your diet. Then you'll no longer be a slave to sugar.

WHOA

MEAT PHYSICALLY MADE TO EAT

TRUE/WERE BIOLOGICALLY

NOT BIOLOGICALLY/NOT

Lie #2: The U.S. Department of Agriculture Knows What Should Be on Your Plate

Surely you knew there'd be a second lie.

You know by now that sugar has been pumped into the
food chain over the last fifty years, especially in the form of
high-fructose corn syrup (HFCS). As a result, there has been
a dramatic increase in a whole range of illnesses that manifest
in different parts of your bodies, depending on your own
genetic profile. All are caused by the same underlying impact

---

*Without this evolutionary mechanism, our primordial ancestors would
have exploded their guts in times of feasting. Sound familiar? And the
same is true of all mammals.

of inflammation from sugar, and the resulting nerve damage and compression. Medical professionals can be blinded by the bias of their specialties and miss the important connections linking these seemingly unrelated conditions. But like us, they're hampered by information linked to the partnership between the U.S. Department of Agriculture (USDA) and the Big Agra complex.

When the Government Took an Interest in What You Eat

In 1916, the USDA began a well-intended nutrition education program consisting of two publications, "Food for Young Children" and "How to Select Food." These plans established guidelines for groups and households to provide "protective foods." Then, in 1992, after several successive programs, the USDA established the familiar Food Guide Pyramid, with its six basic food groups. The base of the pyramid, as we all recall, consisted of the Bread, Cereal, Rice & Pasta Group. Americans were advised that in order to be healthy, they needed to consume 6–11 servings of these foods per day! The pyramid then stacked foods in descending importance: fruits and vegetables, meats and dairy products, and finally, fats and sweets to be used sparingly. A modified MyPyramid Food Guidance System was initiated in 2005; it added the concept of exercise and stressed moderation in food choices rather than specific daily servings.

The latest incarnation, established in 2011, is a dinner plate icon called MyPlate, which advises us on the percentages of foods we should consume daily: 30 percent grains, 40 percent vegetables, 10 percent fruits, and 20 percent protein, with a small, side portion of dairy.

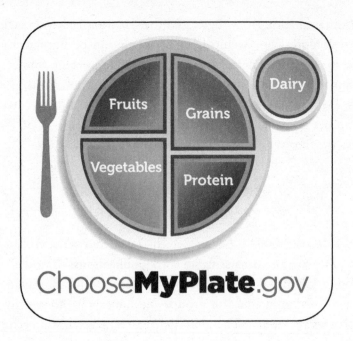

And yet the official government dietary guidelines for healthy eating are dangerously wrong in almost every respect. Like the old food pyramid in its various incarnations, the new food plate is the product of the marriage of politics and Big Agra lobbying—actual nutrition has very little to do with the recommendations. As they stand today, and have for decades, the official recommendations of the USDA are determined by the commercial interests of agribusiness. They're also the primary reason why two-thirds of all Americans are overweight. They're why 29 million Americans have type 2 diabetes, another 19 million have it but don't know it, and 79 million people have prediabetes. They're also why I never lack for patients suffering from diabetic peripheral neuropathy.

So, what's wrong with MyPlate? Almost everything. Specifically, the USDA officially promotes a diet that is far too high in carbohydrates and far too low in healthy fat. In other words, your government is promoting a diet that will make you obese, give you a whole slew of illnesses, and kill your nerves.

How Did These Dangerous USDA Recommendations Get Started?

It all started back in the 1950s, when there was an epidemic of middle-aged men dropping dead of heart attacks. The cause, according to the experts, was too much saturated fat in the diet. How did they arrive at this assumption? First, because they knew that a heart attack is caused by a blockage in an artery nourishing the heart. They also knew that atherosclerotic plaques, made up mostly of cholesterol, caused the blockage. And because foods that are high in saturated fat, such as meat, also contain cholesterol, they came to the conclusion, *with very little evidence*, that a high-fat diet caused heart disease.

Much as I like to see dots connected, the steps that link saturated fat in the diet to a higher risk of a heart attack were unproved then—and they remain unproved. Even so, the saturated fat–cholesterol–heart hypothesis became an article of faith.

But was there actually an epidemic of heart attacks among middle-aged men in the 1950s? No. Instead, there was an epidemic of men aged 50 and up. In 1900, the average life expectancy of an American male was 48 years. Most men died of infectious diseases such as tuberculosis, pneumonia, diphtheria, and gastrointestinal illnesses. Accidents of various sorts killed many more men than they do today. In 1900, nutritional deficiencies were fairly common. Pellagra, caused by a lack of the B vitamin niacin, was widespread in the South until the 1930s and beyond.

By 1950, however, the average American male was living into his seventies. Death from infectious disease was way down, due to improved living conditions and the discovery of antibiotics. Death from malnutrition was rare and overall, life was safer and healthier. Many more men were now making it into their fifties and beyond, reaching the prime heart attack years. That means more men were dying of heart attacks simply because more were surviving long enough to have one.

The apparent increase in the rate of heart attacks got a lot of attention, mostly from older white men who were worried about having one themselves (more women die of heart attacks than men, but that fact was largely ignored in the uproar). Then, when President Dwight David "Ike" Eisenhower had a heart attack in 1955, his cardiologist, the famed Dr. Paul Dudley White, blamed the president's high-fat diet and put him on a low-fat diet instead. (The fact that Eisenhower had smoked four packs of cigarettes a day up until 1949 didn't seem to cross anyone's mind as being a likely cause.) When Ike ran again for president in 1956, the low-fat diet was credited for his recovery and ability to return to work. What never got publicized is that Ike hated his low-fat diet. He felt hungry all the time even as he gained weight and his cholesterol continued to rise. He also continued to have heart attacks—six more after leaving office. The last and fatal attack occurred in 1969.

Again, Follow the Money

The supposed link between saturated fats and heart disease was a marketing windfall for the food industry. Suddenly they had a demand for a product that had been pretty un-popular up until then: margarine. In the 1860s, Emperor Napoleon II of France offered a prize for anyone who could come up with an acceptable substitute for butter. Because butter is made from milk, and because cows go dry in the winter, butter in those days before refrigeration was a scarce and expensive commodity. Also, because butter was made by hand on the farm, the quality varied and dairy farmers and retailers were tempted to cheat by adulterating the butter with colorings and flavorings. The prize was won in 1869 by a French chemist named Hippolyte Mège-Mouriès. Alas, the next year saw the outbreak of the Franco-Prussian War and Napoleon's abdication; his margarine process, which used beef tallow, never got the government backing Mège-Mouriès hoped for and he died in poverty in 1880.

When hydrogenation, which converts liquid vegetable oils into soft solids, was invented in the early 1900s, margarine became cheaper and easier to produce. It continued to be sold as a cheap substitute for butter, but it was strongly opposed by the dairy industry, for obvious reasons. The industry particularly objected to the use of yellow dye to make the unattractive white margarine look even more tempting than real butter.* Margarine gradually caught on as a cheap butter substitute, even though it didn't really taste much like butter. However, when the saturated fat in butter was named public enemy number one for heart disease, margarine began to be touted as a healthier substitute.

---

*Some states actually banned dyed margarine, and for years the package contained a little packet of dye that the purchaser would mix in to make the margarine look as yellow as she liked.

What could be better from a marketing standpoint? Concerned housewives bought margarine to save their husbands from a heart attack—and saved money at the same time! There was just one catch. The manufacturing process that made margarine solid at room temperature did so by changing the molecular structure of the fat molecules. They were warped into something called *trans fatty acids*, or trans fats for short. Nobody knew it at the time, but trans fats are the only kind of fat that is genuinely bad for your health. Unlike other forms of fat, trans fats have been conclusively shown to contribute to heart disease and diabetes. For decades, the American public was completely duped into eating something that was actually more harmful than what it replaced.

Something very similar happened with lard, once a staple fat for cooking. Scarcity, expense, and adulteration were problems with lard. When a solid white shortening known as Crisco became available in 1911, it caught on quickly.* That it, like margarine, was very high in trans fats wasn't seen as a problem until decades later.

And then a highly respected researcher named Ancel Keys said that he *had proved* the link from saturated fat to heart disease based on his study of the diets of people in seven countries around the world.

The Seven Countries Study

During World War II, Ancel Keys was the researcher who worked out the nutritional requirements for soldiers in the

---

*For one thing, Crisco was easy to work with and made the absolutely *best* pie crust. Many people growing up in the 1950s and '60s came to think of Crisco as "healthy lard."

field.* K rations weren't all that successful taste-wise, as anyone who had to eat them would tell you; but they were widely credited with keeping GIs in the field well fed, strong, and ready to fight.

After the war, Dr. Keys turned his attention to heart disease. He thought that high cholesterol levels were a good predictor of heart disease and that dietary fat, especially the saturated fat found in animal foods such as meat and cheese, was bad for the heart. To prove his point, he became the lead researcher in a massive study of dietary patterns around the world that came to be called the Seven Countries Study. This study, begun in 1955, put the American diet onto the misguided path we're still on today. Although Dr. Keys had the best of intentions and didn't have the industry ties so many scientists have today, his work fed right into the hands of Big Agra and Big Pharma.

Ancel Keys sent everyone's focus off in the wrong direction. The pharmaceutical companies and the USDA capitalized on this, and the result is that Americans are fat. Not because they're eating fat, but because they aren't. This is an extremely important point, but most of my patients don't get it. Many of my patients don't understand that their weight problems and illnesses are caused not by the fat in their diets but by the massive amounts of sugar and unrefined carbs they eat. They've been told for so long that fat is bad that they simply take it for granted as true.

---

*Legend has it that this is the origin of the term K-rations. In reality, the letter *K* was chosen to distinguish the rations from earlier versions. I've often wondered if Dr. Keys was also responsible for the decision to include four cigarettes in each package. If so, he was a lot more responsible for heart attacks in the 1950s than any of his nutritional suspects.

The Seven Countries Study is considered a landmark in nutrition. It's the study that "proved" the link between a high-fat diet and heart disease. The goal of the study was to look at the diets of different populations around the world and discover how diet affected heart disease. By comparing the health of groups of middle-aged men in each country over time, Keys hoped to discover the underlying dietary components that led to, or prevented, heart disease.

It took until 1970 for the results to start appearing. When they did, they seemed to prove the fat diet–heart hypothesis. Deaths from heart attacks were low in Crete, where the population ate little meat, and high in countries like Finland and the United States. Keys drew three conclusions from the study. First, he said it proved that high cholesterol levels predicted heart disease. Second, he said it proved that a diet high in saturated fat raised cholesterol levels and therefore predicted heart disease. And finally, he said he had proof that monounsaturated fats (the kind in vegetable oil) helped protect against heart disease.

There was one big problem with the Seven Countries Study, however—Keys cherry-picked the populations studied. He knew from earlier work that the countries he chose would support his hypothesis. Over the years, another big problem became clear. The data Keys collected didn't support his conclusions. High cholesterol did mean a higher rate of heart disease, for example; but overall, the populations in the study who ate the most saturated fat lived longer than those who ate less. American men, who ate a lot of saturated fat, had longer life expectancies than did Japanese men, who ate far less.

As the best hucksters know, never let the facts get in the way of a good story. The idea that saturated fat was bad for you was intuitively satisfying. After all, if you pour bacon fat down the drain you'll clog it up. Wouldn't it be the same for your arteries? And in the late 1960s and early 1970s, the renowned Dr. Keys was supposedly proving that fat was bad for you.

His contention was bolstered by early results from the Framingham Heart Study, which started in 1948. The study followed the heart health of residents in Framingham, Massachusetts, over time—in fact, the study is still running and now includes grandchildren of the original participants. In 1961, the Framingham study reported that high cholesterol levels were associated with a higher risk of heart disease. Later studies in the 1960s and 1970s cited other risk factors for heart disease, such as cigarette smoking, high blood pressure, stress, and obesity. The studies also showed that exercise lowers the risk of heart disease.

There is a significant gap in the logic at the core of these recommendations. None of the research that supposedly supports the recommendations provides any evidence that cutting saturated fat or cholesterol from the diet has any impact at all on coronary heart disease (the kind that gives you a heart attack). And in all the years since then, the huge number of studies on the saturated fat–heart link have still not proved a connection.

Flawed Government Guidelines

That brings our story up to 1976 and the birth of official government guidelines for healthy eating. The Dietary Guidelines for Americans had their start in hearings held by Senator George McGovern's Select Committee on Nutrition and Human Needs. This is the committee that looked into the serious problem of hunger in America and brought landmark legislation, such as the food stamp program, to the nation. As the committee's work drew to an end, staffers decided to look at the other side of the issue: overnutrition and the role of diet in disease. Based on expert testimony from nutritionists who were convinced of the saturated fat–heart hypothesis, in 1977 the committee issued dietary recommendations that pushed for a sharp reduction in fat intake. They recommended limiting total fat intake to 30 percent of calories, of which no more than 10 percent should come from saturated fat. At that time, most Americans got about 40 percent of their calories from fat.

The recommendations ignited a firestorm of controversy. Because a good way to cut fat in the diet is to eat less meat and dairy products, the cattle and dairy industries were furious. So were other segments of Big Agra, such as the manufacturers of vegetable oils and shortenings. The idea that Americans should ever eat *less* of anything incited every agricultural and food processing lobbyist in the country to protest.

In response to the pressure, the guidelines compromised on the dietary fat recommendations, but they still strongly suggested cutting back. The McGovern committee closed down as scheduled in 1979. The dietary guidelines recommendations, rather than expiring with the committee, ended up being taken on by the USDA, where they have remained ever since.

Every five years since the late 1970s, the USDA has issued a set of dietary guidelines for Americans. And every five years, predictably, the food industry rises up to make sure that eating less of anything isn't in those guidelines. Politics and lobbying shape these dietary recommendations far more than actual science.

Not coincidentally, the surge in weight gain among Americans that had begun with the introduction of high-fructose corn syrup gathered steam with the introduction of the food pyramid and its emphasis on carbohydrates. It's not that many adults deliberately followed the pyramid guidelines, because most didn't. Overall, our consumption of fruits and vegetables didn't increase, and while our fat consumption dropped, it never approached the 30 percent of calories in the recommendations. Today, after decades of dietary advice, scarcely one in ten Americans eats four servings of fresh vegetables a day. Most eat barely one—the lettuce and tomato that come on a fast-food burger.

The really insidious part of the guidelines is that they're the standard used for school nutrition programs, for nutritional support programs such as WIC and SNAP, and for meal planning in nursing homes and other institutions—in other words, for any food program that involves government money. That's why your child can be served potato chips in the school lunch program and have them count as a vegetable, or be given a glass of orange juice (another name for concentrated sugar) and have it count as a fruit. It's also why milk, which is high in sugar in the form of lactose, and flavored yogurt, containing both lactose and added sugar, are pushed in school cafeterias. In other words, official government nutrition recommendations lay the groundwork for later nerve damage.

What About USDA Serving Recommendations?

When we look at the serving recommendations issued by the USDA, we can see yet again how the official dietary guidelines contribute to everything wrong with the American diet. Let's take them food group by food group:

- **Fruits**. The recommendation is for 1.5 to 2 cups of fruit or fruit juice daily. Not bad, perhaps even on the low side for someone without blood sugar issues—except that 8 ounces of 100 percent fruit juice counts as a serving. This is the equivalent of swallowing down four teaspoons of sugar at once, a good way to spike your blood sugar even if you don't have prediabetes or diabetes. Also, fruit cocktail or canned fruit in sugary syrup counts as a serving.

- **Vegetables**. The recommendation is for 2 to 3 cups daily. You'd never know it from looking at the MyPlate graphic, which shows vegetables filling a quarter of the plate, but the actual recommendation is for filling half your plate with vegetables at each meal. Again, not bad, but there's a huge problem with this recommendation: potatoes, which are almost pure carbohydrate, are considered a vegetable. Given that Americans consume vast quantities of potatoes, mostly in the form of French fries (29 pounds of fries a year for the average person), this recommendation is practically a prescription for obesity, diabetes, and nerve damage.

- **Proteins**. The recommendation is for 5 to 6.5 ounces daily. The food sources in this category include meat, poultry, fish, and eggs, along with beans and nuts—not so different from earlier recommendations. The problem? While those healthy beans, peas, and lentils are good sources of plant protein, they also contain lots of carbohydrates. One cup of cooked kidney beans, for instance, has about 13 grams of protein—and 38 grams of carbohydrates. Your nerves aren't going to be helped by swapping steak for beans.

- **Dairy products**. The recommendation is for 3 cups a day of preferably low-fat products from this group. One cup of milk, no matter how much fat it has, contains about 11 grams of carbohydrates, mostly in the form of lactose, or milk sugar. Skim milk is really *scam* milk. They took the fat out, which is what you need; and left the sugar in, which is the real problem. Once again, you're being told to eat or drink too much sugar.

- **Grains**. The recommendation is for 3 to 4 ounces a day. Of those, half should be whole grain. Three to 4 ounces doesn't seem like that much. In fact, for someone with normal blood sugar, it isn't—if you understand that a single slice of bread or half a cup of cooked rice or pasta counts as a portion. That part, like all portion sizes, is buried several layers down on the MyPlate website. Very, very few people actually stick to the limited amount of grains in the recommendations. And as I mentioned before, it's also very difficult to eat genuine whole grains. Most of the so-called whole-wheat bread sold in the supermarket is nothing but white flour dyed brown and each slice contains a hefty dose of high-fructose corn syrup.

What have we learned from dissecting the food plate guidelines? That distorted reasoning tilts them heavily toward sugar. According to the guidelines, a lunch that consisted of a cheeseburger on a white bun with lettuce and tomato, a large order of fries, a big glass of fruit juice, and sweetened yogurt for dessert would put you halfway toward meeting your daily nutritional recommendations for a healthy diet. Or, from another point of view, it would put you another step further down the road to neuropathy, disability, and amputation.

YOU'VE GOT TO BE KIDDING

The Missing Animal Proteins

Here's what nearly always happens when I say to my patients, "Tell me about your diet." They lean in and say knowingly, "I don't eat any red meat." The inference is that they're not eating red meat, so they're not eating fat and they think that is good. In fact, they have been dutiful by following the misguided food pyramid recommendations to not eat fat. When I tell them that even though they've been following the rules, the rules are wrong, they're usually frustrated and angry. How could they have actually been hurting themselves? How could they have been duped by this? They believed the government's recommendations and are indignant that they've been badly misinformed for so many years.

Time to Take Action

It's not too late to steer your diet in the right direction. You now know that, regardless of government dietary guidelines, your focus should be on a diet high in grass-fed animal fat and low in sugar and carbohydrates. Chapter 10 will show you how to achieve this diet. But before you move on, take a moment to reflect on the following three profiles of neuropathy:

No !!!

1. **Beginning Stage**. You have a family history of diabetes, but no symptoms yet. And you're in one of the under-40 age demographics. If you stop all sugar now, you can increase not only your quality of life, but quantity of life as well.

2. **Mid-Stage**. You've enjoyed a lifetime of sweets, salty carbs, and the demon rum, but it's beginning to take its toll. It's harder to lose weight; you wake with aches and pains; your blood pressure is rising. You can still prevent significant damage to your end organs, thus extending life to your genetic timetable.

3. **End Stage**. Cutting sugar now can ease your pain and significantly increase your quality of life.

While you may have read thus far because of concern for someone else—a parent, husband, or best friend—it's more likely you've come to recognize *yourself* in one of these profiles. The good news is that cutting sugar from your diet can help, no matter what stage you're in. And it's time to revise our diets so that we're helping ourselves, not hurting ourselves.

10

So Then What Can You Eat?

HOT BUTTERED COFFEE

with Judy Nicassio

What did you eat yesterday? Chances are you started with some sort of breakfast cereal or bread, maybe last night's kung pao; perhaps you had pancakes or a toaster pastry with a glass of OJ. At your morning coffee break, you had a doughnut, or a strawberry muffin, plus a coffee with sugar and milk. At lunch, you ate a sandwich with chips and coleslaw; or perhaps a burger or a burrito; or maybe some pizza, with a dutiful side salad. For your afternoon break, you had cheese crackers from a vending machine; then there was a promotion celebration at the office and you ate a little cake. For dinner, a big plate of pasta—whole wheat to make it healthier—followed by a bowl of ice cream with a chocolate-dipped biscotti. Later, while watching a movie, you had some microwave popcorn. The fat-free kind.

In other words, like most Americans, you primarily ate highly processed carbohydrates. That means you also ate a

lot of sugar. Is it any mystery why you've been slowly putting on weight around your waistline? And is it any wonder
you've been having headaches, stomach pains that come and
go, aching and tingling in your feet and legs, an annoying
case of carpal tunnel syndrome in your wrist, and a variety
of zings and zaps in other joints?

I want to give you two methods for radically improving
your health and healing your nerves.

Your Food Path to Health and Pain Relief

Personally, I follow a strict *ketogenic* diet, which involves
eating very low to zero carbohydrates, a moderate amount
of grass-fed animal protein, and a predominant amount
of grass-fed fats (including butter, hard and soft cheeses,
and real cream). An easy way to think of it is halting your
consumption of all sugar, processed foods, and hidden
carbohydrates—cold turkey. In the pages that follow, this
ketogenic approach will be labeled Plan A.

However, many of my patients find Plan A difficult
to sustain, and so I asked a nutritionist, Judy Nicassio, to
devise an alternate approach allowing you to also taper off
carbohydrates and bring your body's chemistry back into
its normal, healthful state. I'll call that Plan B. Based on the
glycemic index and adapted from food options developed by
Dr. Joseph Mercola and others, Judy calls this program the
Blood Sugar Regulation Diet and it includes limited dairy
and a variety of fruits and vegetables with low to moderate
glycemic levels. The choice is yours.

Both plans require you to remove *all* processed foods,
table sugar, and artificial sweeteners from your diet and are
thus *anti-inflammatory*. Importantly, both will help ease

your neuropathic pain and are associated with many health benefits as well, including lowered blood pressure, weight loss, lowered triglycerides, increased mental clarity, physical energy, improved immunity, and resolution of digestive tract disorders including irritable bowel syndrome.

Of course, as with all things in life, we must be mindful before undertaking change. Low-carb/high-protein/high-fat diets can be contraindicated for some individuals including: women who are nursing or pregnant, women with fertility complications, athletes requiring high glycolytic output, and individuals with kidney disease, hypothyroidism, or adrenal fatigue. And if you already have diabetes and are taking medications for various conditions, such as high blood pressure or cholesterol, have a serious discussion with your physician regarding what you've learned about the catastrophic effects of sugar. Be your own advocate and ask how you can wean yourself off pharmaceuticals.

Regardless of whichever plan you choose, I recommend starting the day with hot buttered coffee.

Hot Buttered Coffee

Often when I recommend a morning cup of hot buttered coffee I'll get a response such as "Yuck!" And yet, when this same person tries it, he's likely to come back a true convert. This is because starting your day with hot buttered coffee has three amazing effects:

- First, it gives you a steady energy level that lasts for hours. You won't get that from sugary breakfast cereal (especially the ones touting they are fat-free/heart healthy), OJ, or toaster pastries—in fact, just the opposite. Most people are quickly hungry again after starting the day with sugar.

- Second, hot buttered coffee suppresses your appetite. You won't want a snack at morning break time and you'll probably eat less at lunch.
- Third, when you limit your diet to just fats (the true ketogenic state), drinking hot buttered coffee will produce a one-pound-a-day loss in weight.

Even if you already use milk or cream, the idea of putting butter in your coffee can seem strange; and yet butter is more flavorful. More important, making this your morning beverage is a great way to start your day with a big dose of healthy fat.

One tablespoon of butter (one-eighth of a stick) has about 11 grams of fat, as compared to 5 grams in heavy cream and only half a gram in whole milk. You consume approximately 100 calories from a tablespoon of butter, and, of course, no calories from the coffee. This equals calories of pure energy. Compare that to coffee with two tablespoons of milk (18 calories) and one teaspoon of sugar (16 calories). How can a drink with 34 calories be worse than one with 100? Easy, because butter has no carbohydrates—it doesn't trigger the same spike-and-crash insulin response you get when adding sugar and milk (to say nothing of nonfat, HFCS half-and-half). And it tastes great—creamy, not greasy.

Hot buttered coffee is sometimes called bulletproof coffee. There are plenty of elaborate recipes for it on the Web, but I like to keep things simple. Just put a tablespoon-sized glob of unsalted organic butter in the bottom of your mug. Don't use any other kind of butter, because you want the extra omega-3 fatty acids in the organic. Add hot coffee; let it sit for about fifteen seconds to melt the butter; then stir it up and enjoy. If you want to avoid caffeine, decaffeinated coffee works just as well. Interestingly, however, my caffeine-sensitive patients tell me that when they add butter to regular coffee, they don't feel their normal caffeine jitters.*

General Misconceptions About Coffee

When I extol the virtues of hot buttered coffee, I find many people are often confused about coffee in general. They vaguely think that coffee is just bad for you, or that it causes heart disease (no evidence for this even if you drink six cups a day), or they're concerned about the caffeine (for whatever reason.) A ten-year follow-up of almost 86,000 women in the United States, ages 34–59 and without history of coronary heart disease (CHD), concluded, "These data indicate that coffee as consumed by US women is not an important cause of CHD." While it's true that caffeine can cause wakefulness or keep you from falling asleep, and that the dose of caffeine in a cup of strong coffee does cause a small, temporary rise in blood pressure, coffee has numerous beneficial effects. It seems to help prevent some chronic illness, such as Parkinson's disease, and also may protect against gallstones and liver cancer.

Several studies over the years support the idea that coffee can actually help prevent diabetes. In 2014, researchers at the Harvard School of Public Health looked at the coffee-drinking habits of participants in the long-running Nurses' Health Study, the follow-up Nurses' Health Study II, and the Health Professionals Follow-up Study—a total of more than 125,000

---

*Tea lovers can try this as well. In Tibet, tea made with yak butter and salt is a favorite drink.

CANCER : COFFEE BEANS WHEN HEATED

men and women. The researchers found that over a four-year period, those who increased their coffee consumption by more than one cup a day saw their risk of type 2 diabetes drop by 11 percent, compared to those who made no changes in their coffee consumption. The participants who drank the most coffee—more than three cups a day—had a 37 percent lower risk of diabetes. Those who cut their coffee consumption over the four-year period saw their risk of type 2 diabetes *increase* by 17 percent. The effect seems to come from the coffee itself, not the caffeine. Decaf coffee had the same impact.*

What is it in coffee that provided the protection? It could be that coffee is a good source of magnesium, and to some degree, potassium and niacin as well. Or maybe it's the *polyphenols* in coffee, which are powerful antioxidants; or perhaps some other compound altogether. When I look at the various coffee/diabetes studies, I'm struck by something the researchers never seem to mention: people who drink more coffee probably also drink fewer sugary beverages, such as orange juice or soda. In addition to getting the benefits of the coffee itself, the coffee also displaces sugar water from their diets. That would certainly cut the risk of diabetes. Whatever it is, if you're at risk for diabetes or already have it, I strongly recommend drinking a couple of cups of coffee or more every day.

There is one slight drawback to increased coffee consumption. If you already have diabetes, drinking the equivalent of two cups of strong coffee (about 250 mg of caffeine) could cause a small, temporary rise in your blood sugar. This seems

---

*Tea drinkers who drank more than three or four cups a day had about a 20 percent lower risk of diabetes.

to be because the caffeine increases insulin resistance. Is this enough to make a real difference to you? Probably not, especially if you use hot buttered coffee as a way to avoid eating other sugar and refined carbohydrates, which raise your blood sugar much more and for longer. If this is a concern, simply switch to decaf.

Give hot buttered coffee a try. If it's not for you, no problem. Bacon and eggs with plenty of butter works just as well.

What to Eat the Rest of the Day

Plan A: The Ketogenic Diet

In 1931, the physiologist Otto Warburg won the Nobel Prize for research into cellular respiration showing that cancers thrive in anaerobic (without oxygen) or acidic environments. His conclusions that cancer cells can grow in an abundance of glucose and that *ketones*, the by-product of burning fat for energy, killed cancer cells remained controversial for almost eight decades. However, researchers building on the Warburg effect, as it's called, came to believe that a *ketogenic diet*, one that contains very little sugar or carbohydrates, can effectively treat cancer. This works because healthy cells in the body can burn either glucose or ketones, the fuel made when body fat is broken down for energy.* Cancer cells can only

---

*You may have heard the term *ketosis*. This is a metabolic state in which fat is burned off at a rapid rate. Ketosis can be monitored with reagent strips that register ketones in urine—and some of my patients cite these as good behavioral modification tools. An often cited clinical signal of ketosis is "bad breath." It's important for your physician to periodically monitor ketosis for possible *ketoacidosis*, an extremely rare condition in which abnormal quantities of ketones are produced.

use glucose and if they're starved of it, they die. Moreover, if you don't produce excess insulin to handle excess glucose, you starve the cancer cells even faster.*

So essentially, the ketogenic approach to cancer turns the cancer cells' own metabolism against them. A ketogenic diet is at least 75 percent fat and limits carbs to under 50 grams a day. It can be a hard diet to follow, but it's doable. For example, in the early 1900s, a Harvard study on the traditional Inuit diet showed that their diet was essentially fat. Despite that, they had very little evidence of the Western lifestyle diseases we've been talking about. More recent studies have focused on the extremely low levels of cardiovascular disease, high blood pressure, and cholesterol among the Maasai, the pastoral tribe living in northern Tanzania and Kenya, who have traditionally eaten an exclusive diet of milk, blood, and meat,† which is rich in lactose, fat, and cholesterol. And yet the studies' conclusions focus on the specifics of genetic homogeneity, rather than the inherent value in the high-fat diet itself.

Interestingly, a ketogenic diet has been known since the 1920s to be very helpful for some types of epilepsy. It's considered standard care, even though nobody really knows for certain why it works. We are sure why a ketogenic diet can help stop or slow the spread of cancer, but it's still thought to be a very fringe treatment that no doctor should recommend.

Fortunately, some serious studies of the diet are finally under way, so it's possible the ketogenic approach will

---

*Interestingly, it is reputed that by the time Dr. Warburg reached the end of his life in 1970, he had become so fearful of processed and cancer-enhancing foods that he ate only organic bread and butter.

†With the occasional bit of honey beer, usually reserved for ceremonies and honored guests.

become more mainstream as the positive results are published. We already know from a small study of ten patients with advanced bladder cancer that just four weeks on a ketogenic diet helped stabilize the disease or put it into partial remission in six of the ten cases. That's an encouraging result.

In 2012, a team led by Adrienne C. Scheck, Ph.D., principal investigator in neuro-oncology and neurosurgery research at Barrow Neurological Institute in Phoenix, Arizona, effectively treated brain tumor cells in mice using a combination of a ketogenic diet and radiation therapy. One theory as to why this was successful is that the ketogenic diet may inhibit the growth of tumors by reducing growth factor stimulation. Another theory says that the ketogenic diet may also reduce inflammation and swelling from fluids surrounding the tumors.

If high blood sugar markedly increases your risk of cancer, does getting your blood sugar down reduce it? That's hard to say with certainty because cell changes that cause cancer begin years, sometimes decades, before the cancer becomes evident. The damage from years of high blood sugar and high insulin can't necessarily be overcome or stopped if you get those levels down. On the other hand, we know that a good diet, physical activity, and weight loss all reduce risk and improve outcomes for some forms of cancer, so it's never too late. In my own practice, I see that patients who immediately stop eating all sugars become healthier overall—the benefits aren't just to their feet.

My Green-Yellow-Red Fat Rule

Making high-fat/ketogenic food choices can be daunting, whether at home, a restaurant, in the grocery, or at social events. So I've developed an easy-to-remember mnemonic device for ranking fats and staying on track. I call it the Green-Yellow-Red Fat Rule and here's how it works:

GREEN—Go for it. Any fat product from animals that eat grass is good: meat, eggs, butter, and fish oil.* Additionally, meat and eggs from organically raised grass-fed animals are naturally higher in healthier, *anti-inflammatory* omega-3 fatty acids.† Eat as many of these foods as you like—because as they keep you satiated, you'll shortly discover that you won't want to eat the quantities you once did.

YELLOW—Yellow represents any fat from a grain-fed animal. And although these cautionary foods are sometimes allowed, they're not going to be as healthy for you as grass-fed because they contain a disproportionate amount of the *pro-inflammatory* omega-6 fatty acids.

RED—Red represents trans-fatty acids: artificially produced hydrogenated oils. *Do not eat* these fats in any form. Ever. Your body doesn't have the enzymes necessary to process and eliminate them. Period.

Plan B: The Blood Sugar Regulation Diet

There are two ways to reduce sugar and avoid damage to your nerves: eat more fat and choose carbohydrates that have both a low *glycemic index* and a low *glycemic load*. Such foods will have the least impact on your blood sugar.

---

*Most fish generally eat algae, plankton, or other fish that eat such things.

†Remember the discussion of lesser omega-6s and better omega-3s in the previous chapter. Researchers at North Dakota State University found that while grass-fed bison meat had an omega 6–omega-3 ratio of 4:1, grain-fed bison had a ratio of 21:1, more than 5 times omega-3s in grass-fed animals.

The Glycemic Index

The glycemic index (GI), in particular, takes the guesswork out of the process and many helpful books and websites list the rankings for a wide range of food choices. Developed by nutrition researchers in the 1990s as a way to help people with diabetes, it's become a very helpful and popular guide for anyone looking to cut sugar in her diet. The GI is a powerful tool for understanding how quickly the sugar or other carbohydrates in sugary or starchy plant foods are converted to glucose and absorbed into your bloodstream.

The scientific purpose of the glycemic index is to compare the ability of different carbohydrate-rich foods to raise your blood sugar and your insulin level. Because foods with a high GI value almost always contain a lot of sugar or *refined carbs*, they are absorbed into the bloodstream quickly and can cause a dramatic rise in blood sugar and a spike in insulin production. We can think of these foods as *high-glycemic carbs*. Foods with medium or low GI values that are made up of complex carbs have much less of an impact.

In the glycemic index, carbohydrate-containing foods are ranked by comparing them either to a standard amount of pure glucose or to a slice of white bread. The glucose level of white bread is ranked at 100. Eat pure glucose or white bread and the glucose will enter your blood almost at once. Eat a serving of kidney beans, however, and the carbs will be converted to blood sugar much more slowly. Why? The glucose in beans is tied up with plant fiber. And so, because it takes more time to digest beans enough to release glucose, it enters your bloodstream much more slowly and steadily. Careful research has put a number on approximately how fast the glucose from kidney beans hits your bloodstream, and on the glycemic index, kidney beans are ranked at 23.

The essence of what makes a food rank low on the GI index is the amount of indigestible plant parts it contains. Fiber is what gives celery its crunch and an apple its snap. Fiber slows down the digestion of the food, which in turn means the carbs reach your blood sugar later rather than sooner. And because the difference between high-GI and low-GI foods lies mostly in how much fiber each contains, we need only look at the way fiber is removed from modern-day processed foods (where most of the other nutrients are removed as well) to recognize the lost benefits. The more highly processed a food is, the higher its GI rank. The smaller the starchy particles in the food (think McDonald's hamburger rolls versus grainy pumpernickel bread), the faster those carbs are absorbed and thus the higher the GI value. A slice of commercial whole wheat bread has a GI value of 72, while by comparison, a spoonful of white table sugar has a GI value of 59.

GI Rankings

1. A GI rank of 70 or more is considered to be high;
2. A GI rank of 56–69 is medium; and
3. A GI rank of 55 or less is low.

As a rule of thumb, any food with a GI rank below 55 is a *very* good choice because in addition to being low in calories, it's also likely to be high in vitamins, minerals, and fiber—so its sugar and nutrients will enter your bloodstream slowly.

Many vegetables are very low in carbs and rank zero on the GI scale. These include broccoli, cabbage, cauliflower, cucumber, green beans, and leafy greens (spinach, chard, kale, lettuce, and other salad greens). Generally speaking, starchier foods such as grains and potatoes are higher on the GI scale; most fruit falls below the starchy foods but above the veggies.

The Glycemic Load

The GI value of a food indicates only how quickly a standard amount of carbohydrate, usually 35 or 50 grams, is absorbed into your bloodstream. The calculation is based on an amount of the food that's large enough to contain 35 or 50 grams of carbohydrate. For foods that are lower on the GI ranking, that often works out to be much more food than you would normally eat. In some cases, such as carrots or parsnips, this means the GI value is misleadingly high. To help people use the glycemic index rankings to make good food choices, the researchers came up with the idea of the *glycemic load* (GL). The GL of a food is based on how much of the carbohydrate is digested (available) in *a standard serving* of a particular food. (In case you're interested, the GL is calculated by taking the GI value as a percentage and multiplying by the amount of net carbohydrates—the carbohydrates minus the indigestible fiber.) So, for example, the kidney beans I mentioned above have a GI of 23. But if you eat a standard serving of about two-thirds of a cup of kidney beans, you get only 17 grams of carbs, for a glycemic load of 8. A more dramatic example is watermelon, which has a high GI of 72. But in a standard 4-ounce serving, there are only 6 grams of available carbs, which works out to a low glycemic load ranking of 4. Likewise for parsnips, which are often shunned for having a high GI ranking of 97. (Okay, there may be other reasons to shun parsnips.) On the GL scale, however, parsnips are ranked at 10. Why the difference? Parsnips are relatively high in fiber, which slows the entry of glucose into the blood.

GL Rankings

1. A GL ranking of 20 or more is high.
2. A GL ranking of 11–19 is medium; and
3. A GL ranking of 10 or less is low.

Because the glycemic load is based on normal portion sizes, it is a more realistic measure of how a food is likely to affect your insulin levels and blood sugar.

Foods for Your Improved Health and Nerves

Appropriate foods for the Blood Sugar Regulation Diet are organized in two charts, Primary and Cautionary (secondary) categories. As you approach the plan, remember the following five easy steps:

1. PRIMARY proteins should be approximately 3–6 ounces per meal. Low-starch foods on the primary list can amount to what fits in a medium-sized bowl.
2. For the first two weeks, eat only *three* ½-cup servings of the CAUTIONARY foods.
3. For the next two weeks, eat only *two* ½-cup servings of the CAUTIONARY foods.
4. For the following two weeks, eat only *one* ½-cup serving of the CAUTIONARY foods.
5. After week 6, you will be consuming mostly "primary foods" (at least 80 percent of the time). The gradual cutting

back of the higher-glycemic foods is a process to avoid severe withdrawals connected to your sugar addition. Once your blood sugars, insulin levels, weight, metabolic syndrome, etc. have stabilized, you may experiment with how often you can include "secondary foods" in your diet. However, for the rest of your life, you'll need to walk that fine line determining the appropriate macronutrient ratios for your changing needs, and this is where guidance from a nutritionist can be beneficial. But you will be happier and healthier—the best motivation of all.

BLOOD SUGAR REGULATION DIET—PRIMARY FOODS*

Proteins†			Carbohydrates†			Fats††
Meats/Fowl	**Fish/Seafood**		**Vegetables**			
			Very Low Glycemic	Very Low Glycemic	Low Glycemic	
Beef	Anchovy	Sole	Celery	Lettuce	Broccoli	Olives
Chicken	Caviar	Flounder	Mushrooms	Mesclun or Spring Mix	Broccoli Raabe	Coconut
Organ Meats: Heart, Liver, Kidney, Sweet Breads, Paté	Herring	Cod	Spinach	Purslane	Brussels Sprout	Avocado
	Mussel	White Sea Bass	Asparagus	Cucumber	Kale	
Turkey	Sardine	Tilapia	Cauliflower	Arugula	Parsley	**Fats** ††
	Tuna	Trout	String beans	Beet Greens	Cilantro	Butter
Bacon	Abalone	Scrod		Endive	Dandelion Greens	Cream
Beef	Arctic char	Grouper		Watercress		Ghee
Buffalo	Clam	Haddock			Collard Greens	
Cornish hen	Crab	Halibut		Vegetable Seed Sprouts	Turnip Greens	**Oils**
Duck	Crayfish	Mahi mahi			Mustard Greens	Olive Oil
Goat	Lobster	Sablefish (Black Cod)		Chard	Tomato	Coconut Oil

Goose	Mackerel	Perch		Horseradish	Bell pepper	Macadamia Nut Oil
Goose	Mackerel	Perch		Horseradish	Bell pepper	Macadamia Nut Oil
Ham	Octopus	Red snapper		Radish	Egg Plant	Flax Sceed Oil
Lamb	Oyster	Skate		Cabbage	Onion	Walnut Oil
Ostrich	Salmon	Salmon		Bok Choy (Chinese Cabbage)	Scallion	Pumpkin Seed Oil
Pheasant	Scallop	Catfish		Radicchio	Leek	Sesame Seed Oil
Pork chop	Squid			Seaweeds	Garlic	May add nuts from the Secondary List in moderation.
Quail	Snail	**Eggs & Dairy**			Shallot	
Spare rib	Shrimp	Eggs (whole)			Ginger Root	
Turkey leg & thigh		Cheese†			Fennel	
Veal		Cottage cheese†				
Venison						
Wild game						

* Adapted from Dr. Joseph Mercola. www.mercola.com.

† When possible, proteins and fats should be grass-fed, free-range, and organic. Fish and seafood should be wild caught.

Carbohydrates should be organic.

‡ See the secondary food list for recommendations on dairy.

BLOOD SUGAR REGULATION DIET— SECONDARY/CAUTIONARY FOODS (WHOLE GRAINS)*

Dairy†	Vegetables†		Sweet Fruits‡		Grains	Seeds & Nuts§
Moderate Glycemic	Moderate Glycemic	High Glycemic	Moderate to High Glycemic		High Glycemic	Low Glycemic
			Fresh, raw, and slightly unripe			
			Eat with peel or skin	Eat without peel or skin		
Whole fat (no skim or light)	Carrot	Parsnip			Whole grains only	Unsalted
Milk	Beet	Potato	Blueberry	Orange	Amaranth	Walnut
Kefir	Jicama	Taro	Raspberry	Tangerine	Brown rice	Pumpkin
Plain yogurt	Okra	Sweet potato	Strawberry	Grapefruit	Buckwheat	Flax seed
Sour cream	Zucchini	Yam	Blackberry	Lemon	Corn (on the cob)	Almond
Eliminate pasteurized dairy products.	Yellow squash	Sunchoke (Jerusalem artichoke)	All other berries	Lime	Millet	Sunflower
	Summer squash				Oat	Sesame
Raw dairy is more nutritionally valuable than	Spaghetti squash	Winter squash	Cherry	Pineapple	Quinoa	Brazil
	Kohlrabi		Grape	Papaya	Triticale	Filbert/hazel

pasteurized dairy and is allowable.

Listings for raw dairy in your area, can be found at: www.realmilk.com.

If unavailable, substitute grass-fed or organic dairy.

Turnip	**Legumes**	Persimmon	Mango	Wild Rice	Pecan
Rutabaga	Beans, dry	Apricot	Cherimoya		Pistachio
Pumpkin	Lentils	Peach	Cantaloupe		Pine nuts
Artichoke	Peas, dry	Nectarine	Watermelon and all other melons	**Starchy nut**	Macadamia
Peas		Plum	Banana	Chestnut**	Cashew
		Fig	Kiwi		
		Apple			
		Pear	**Tart Fruits**		
			Pomegranate		
			Cranberry		
			Lemon		
			Lime		

*Adapted from Dr. Joseph Mercola. www.mercola.com.

† Include small amounts of fat.

‡ Fruits and vegetables should be organic.

§ Nuts and seeds should be used in moderation.

** Unlike any other nut, chestnuts are high in both fat and starch.

Whether You Choose Plan A or Plan B

Deciding to remove sugar from your life is an important step forward. Should you decide to go cold turkey or phase into healthy eating, a few constants remain:

1. Give Up Sugary Drinks

Most Americans get about 30 percent of the liquids they consume from carbonated soft drinks—they drink about 45 gallons a year of the stuff. A can of regular soda has about 9 teaspoons of sugar in it. And that's not counting all the fruit juice, sports drinks, energy drinks, and sweetened tea and coffee you drink. It all makes sugar addiction that much harder to kick. I've had patients who cheerfully gave up doughnuts, pasta, chocolate, and other sugary foods, but absolutely refused to give up diet cola. They felt that compared to other foods, it was a harmless, no-calorie pleasure. Once my soda-addicted patients realize that diet soda isn't such a harmless pleasure after all, they can usually manage to cut consumption or give it up entirely.

Real fruit juice is another sugar addiction that's extremely difficult to abandon. After all, every breakfast cereal commercial you've ever seen also has a glass of orange juice somewhere in camera range. Plus, OJ just tastes good. Drinking a glass of any sort of 100 percent fruit juice, however, isn't much better than injecting it into your bloodstream. The sugar in the juice is absorbed almost instantly—that's why the emergency procedure for someone with hypoglycemic shock is to give him orange juice to instantly raise glucose. But if you already *have* high blood sugar, that's the last thing you want to do. Fruit drinks are nothing more than flavored high-fructose corn syrup and should be completely eliminated from your diet.

Sadly, the introduction of the juice box in the 1980s came shortly after the introduction of HFCS and gave a big push to the obesity epidemic that also started then. Suddenly it was easy and cheap to give your kids regular doses of addictive sugar water.

Sports drinks and energy drinks are also a big part of beverage consumption. They're full of sugar, artificial sweeteners, and additives you don't need. Skip them.

2. Limit Fruit

Once in a while, fresh fruit can be a good substitute as you break away from processed sugars. Yes, fruit contains fructose, but in much smaller amounts compared to high-fructose corn syrup. This fructose is also wrapped up in the fiber of the fruit, which means your body needs to digest the fruit for a while before the fructose is released. The fiber in the fruit also slows absorption of the fructose, while helping you feel full. Some tropical fruits, such as mangos and pineapple, are very sweet. Limit how much of those you eat—one serving a day is plenty. Fruit that has been peeled, cooked, and processed (applesauce, for instance) is no longer fruit—it's sugar. Likewise for fruit that has sugar added to it in other ways, such as dried cranberries or canned fruit in syrup.

To really kick your addiction, though, you need to cut back on sweetness, even if it's coming from fruit. Now would be a good time to switch your snacking over to foods that have less of a sugar punch or no sugar at all. Nuts make an excellent choice—they're crunchy and satisfying, plus they give you a lot of great nutrients like magnesium, fiber, and omega-3 fatty acids. Seeds such as sunflower seeds or pumpkin seeds are great as well. Raw vegetables such as carrots, celery, cucumbers, and sliced peppers are great snacks, especially if you have them with a sugar-free dip such as hummus, guacamole, or salsa. Try keeping a bag of baby carrots, already peeled and washed, in the fridge; you can prepare other vegetables in advance as well. For meals, choose sides that have a sweet flavor, like sweet potatoes, or roasted carrots or squash. Candied sweet potatoes are clearly out, but try sprinkling sweet spices such as cinnamon, allspice, nutmeg, or cloves on these foods to bring out their natural sweetness.

3. Use Real Cream, Not Milk

Milk, despite all the advertising about how good it is for you, is filled with sugar. One cup of milk—whole, skim, or 2 percent—has 12 grams of sugar in the form of lactose. Leaving aside that many people can't digest lactose, that's 3 teaspoons of sugar. In fact, once all healthy animal fat is stripped away from milk, the thin, grayish liquid called skim milk is actually just sugar water. And most milk substitutes, such as rice milk, soy milk, and almond milk, contain added sugar. Check the labels and use real cream in your coffee instead.

4. Avoid Soy

Bet you thought soy was a health food. Despite the best efforts of the FDA and marketing departments within Big Agra, there are many nutrition scientists who think the jury is still out regarding this point. In 1999, the FDA allowed manufacturers to claim that low-fat diets also high in soy may reduce the risk of heart disease. However, a 2014 report from the Harvard School of Public Health stated that this ruling was based on assertions coming from preliminary research and that a number of significant studies since "have tempered this finding, as well as those regarding soy's effects on other conditions." Meanwhile, we know that soy contains *phytoestrogens*, which mimic natural estrogen,* not to mention the fact that 90 percent of soybeans grown in America are genetically modified to resist herbicides. As a result, Big Agra farming practices spray soybean fields liberally—and soybeans grown this way contain large residues of the carcinogen *glyphosate*, a major ingredient in Monsanto's Roundup herbicide. Most of us don't eat that many soybeans, but it is the second-largest U.S. crop after corn and is widely used as feed for commercial livestock. It turns up in grain-fed table meat, cooking oil, and processed foods in general (especially those prepared with cooking oil derivatives).

Soy does have nutritional proteins, but even when grown organically it naturally contains numerous *antinutrients* that can result in growth problems in children, interfere with iodine metabolism, disrupt endocrine function, and prevent your red blood cells from properly absorbing and distributing oxygen—to name a few. These negative compounds are mitigated during the fermentation process (as seen in Asian cuisines), but most Westerners consume *unfermented* soy in the form of soy milk, tofu, and soy infant formula.

---

*This is bad news for males, as excess phytoestrogens can lead to testosterone imbalance and low sperm count.

Lying Labels

You can't move forward without all of the information, so you need to learn how to interpret food labels. In addition, building this habit—checking the label—is critical to your new sugar-free life. And there's no doubt we need an easier system for labeling food so that its real contents are transparent. I recently watched a satirical treatment of this issue delivered by John Oliver—he suggested we label processed foods with the epitome of junk food—fluffy, orange Circus Peanuts. One peanut, you're taking some risk; five peanuts, look out.

Seduced and Betrayed

Start by realizing that sugar is everywhere in processed foods, often in hidden form. On the food facts label, the amount of sugar the product contains is given in grams. Metric numbers baffle Americans, a confusion food manufacturers happily exploit so you don't realize how much sugar their products contain. Just remember that 4 grams of sugar in any form is the equivalent of 1 teaspoon. Now check your fridge and pantry for products that contain sugar. Read the ingredients labels—you'll find that a scary 80 percent of the processed foods in your house have added sugar. Throw or give these foods away. Don't eat them.

However, *added* sugar is only the "up-front" part of the story. You can determine *additional/ hidden* sugar in a processed food by looking at the number of carbohydrates listed on the label—then divide that number by 4.

For example, a 6-ounce bottle of Boost (an energy/protein drink like Ensure) is touted as being enriched with fiber, protein, and muscle-building capabilities. All true. But when you look at the label on the back of the bottle, it also lists 21 carbs. So how many teaspoons of sugar does this tiny bottle have? Divide 21 by 4 and the answer is a bit more than 5. *Five* teaspoons of sugar in a 6-ounce bottle of something you may believe is healthful. Would you add 5 teaspoons of sugar to a glass of iced tea? Probably not. And if the manufacturer is proud of the fact that this is an energy drink, why not put a banner on the front of the bottle—"contains 5 teaspoons of sugar"? In every phase of the marketplace, we are being seduced and betrayed.

As you move from refined carbohydrates to better choices, watch out for whole-grain hype. I spend a great deal of time educating my patients about this. Just because the label on the front of the package proclaims that a food is a good source of whole grains and/or fiber doesn't mean you should eat it. It drives me to distraction that Cheerios is allowed to advertise itself as "heart healthy." Check the food facts label and the ingredients list before you buy.

Navigating the Current Waters

The food facts label on a food package is a confusing mass of government-mandated misinformation. Ignore most of it, especially the nonsense about the fat content. Only three pieces of information on the food facts label actually tell you anything useful.

- **Portion size.** The portion size information tells you how many standard portions are contained in the package. Everything on the rest of the label is based on the size of a single portion, not the total amount contained in the package. This is deliberately (in my view) misleading. A 20-ounce bottle of chocolate drink, for instance, contains 2.5

portions, according to the label. That means you need to do some mental arithmetic to figure out how many calories and other stuff is in the whole bottle, because in all like-lihood you're going to drink all of it at once. If you don't realize you have to do the math, you'll think that you're getting far fewer calories than you actually are.

- **Fat.** Ignore this unless the label says the food contains trans fats. If it does, don't eat it.

- **Total carbohydrates.** Now we're finally getting some useful information. Forget the misleading percentage number and look only at the grams per serving. If it has more than 10 grams of carbohydrate per serving, don't eat it. Under the total carbohydrates heading, look next for the dietary fiber per serving. The more fiber, the better—the fiber will slow down how quickly the glucose enters your bloodstream. Finally, look for sugars. If the food has any, it's from added sugar, not what's naturally in the food. Don't eat it.

Ingredients List

You'll get a lot more information about the food you're about to consume from looking at the ingredients list. Here's an easy rule of thumb: If the ingredients list has more than five items, don't eat it—especially if you can't pronounce ingredients like *distilled monoglycerides* (whatever they are) or *butylated hydroxyanisole* (a preservative usually abbreviated as BHA).

The list starts with the ingredient used in the greatest amount by weight in the food; each ingredient after that is listed in descending order. Here's where the whole-grain hype is most obvious. Unless the first ingredient is truly a whole grain, the food isn't a particularly good source. And even if the first ingredient is whole-grain flour, keep reading to make sure that sugar in some form or other hasn't been added.

Some Examples:

1. Your favorite barbecue sauce: the first ingredient is the sweeter than sugar, high-fructose corn syrup.
2. An Atkins peanut butter cup disguised as a healthful snack contains in descending order: *maltitol* (a sugar alcohol sugar substitute that's 70–90 percent sweeter than table sugar.),* *polydextrose* (a synthetic polymer of glucose), and *sucralose* (an artificial sweetener that is not broken down in the human body).
3. Graham crackers—perhaps no greater corruption.†

Label hype isn't limited to just proclaiming on the front label that a food has some so-called healthy ingredients without bothering to mention all the unhealthy ingredients. Hype also comes from other sources, such as the American Heart Association's amazingly misleading Heart-Check certification. If a food package has the AHA heart logo on it, the food is supposedly heart healthy and a good choice. But to get the certification, the food need only be low in cholesterol and fat—and the manufacturer has to be willing to pay hefty fees for the right to participate in deceptive advertising.

---

*A class of carbohydrate that produces a rise in blood glucose that is only slightly smaller than the rise produced by other carbohydrates. Although called "sugar alcohol," it actually does not contain alcohol.

†In 1829, Sylvester Graham, a Presbyterian minister railing against the Industrial Revolution idea of mass-produced bread, developed a whole-grain flour he believed would cleanse body and soul. We're talking about eternal salvation as the prime motivator here. Nabisco appropriated the graham flour concept, adding sugar and bleached flour to create the beloved and now traditional Honey Maid graham cracker.

When the program started in 1995, it led to laughable results, such as the Heart-Check logo on toaster pastries. Today, the program factors in fiber and added sugar, but the logo is still on plenty of highly processed foods that nobody should eat. Don't fall for it.

Also don't fall for the low-fat/no-fat trap. You know by now that dietary fat is good for you and that carbohydrates aren't. Labels that proclaim a product is a low-fat or no-fat version of an existing product are totally misleading. To replace the fat in a food and make it still taste palatable, the manufacturers simply add more sugar. Most of this deceptive labeling is applied to snack foods and other highly processed foods you now want to avoid anyway, but the "no-fat technique" is also commonly used in salad dressings. Just pass these foods by.

There's a much simpler way to know what's in a food. Buy only whole, organic products without added preservatives and colorings. That way you'll have a much better idea of what you're eating. Even with organic foods, however, you need to be careful to avoid sugar. Organic whole-grain pretzels aren't any better for you than plain old pretzels. Sugar is sugar.

A Word About Exercise

Yes.

Do it for many reasons. Every health-care provider will rightly tell you to move every joint every day in range-of-motion activity. Stretching, walking, any exercise you enjoy—all are essential for your well-being. However, when you have peripheral neuropathy, flexing and splaying out your toes yoga-fashion will increase your blood supply—but it won't extinguish the flame in your nerves. For that you must first modify your diet. As the pain subsides, you'll find yourself wanting to be more active.

Inflammatory Foods

Did you know that there are certain foods that can actually promote inflammation in your body? Many chronic diseases such as arthritis, diabetes, obesity, and cancer have been linked to inflammation. Anytime you're suffering with a condition that causes inflammation in any part of your body for a prolonged period of time, you become much more susceptible to disease states. So it would make sense to reduce the intake of these inflammatory foods to protect your overall health.

Foods to Avoid

Any processed, packaged, or prepared foods (including fast foods) that contain sugars, artificial sweeteners, harmful oils, food additives, etc., will all promote inflammation in your body.

- Sugar, in any form, elevates blood glucose levels and triggers the body's inflammatory response. This includes soft drinks, fruit juices, candy, etc.
- Avoid all trans fats or hydrogenated fats like those found in margarine, shortening, baked goods, and other shelf-stable foods. No amount of trans fats should be consumed.
- Fried foods are the absolute pits. French fries, potato chips, onion rings, etc., expose your body to free-radical damage, hastening your demise!
- Dairy products (excluding organic, grass fed, or raw) are inflammatory and loaded with hormones, antibiotics, and other harmful ingredients.

- Wheat and all gluten-containing grains are not only hard to digest, but are acidic and cause inflammation. Better alternatives are quinoa, buckwheat, and amaranth.
- Artificial sweeteners like aspartame (found in NutraSweet and Equal), saccharin, sucralose, etc., have been linked to many serious illnesses.
- Food additives, such as flavor enhancers like MSG, artificial colors, stabilizers, preservatives, anticaking agents, bulking agents, emulsifiers, glazing agents, and thickeners—the list goes on and on. This plethora of artificial ingredients can have dire consequences for your health.
- Cooking oils high in omega-6 fatty acids, including corn, soy, and canola oils, are extremely fragile—when exposed to heat, air, or light, they will go rancid. This translates into free-radical damage and creates inflammation. If lightly sautéing foods on low heat, you can use olive oil. When cooking at medium to high heat or when baking, it's best to use the more stable coconut oil.
- Alcohol is high in sugar and is a burden on the liver. Overconsumption can increase the body's inflammatory response. Eliminate completely or use in moderation.
- Deli meats, sausages, and bacon are preserved with cancer-causing nitrites and nitrates and thus create inflammation. However, there are some healthier brands available that do not contain these carcinogens.

Eating Out

When you're avoiding sugar and carbohydrates, eating out doesn't have to be a problem. That's important, because most of us eat at least one meal away from home almost every day. At any diner or restaurant, you can easily find choices that won't damage your nerves. Asking for extra veggies or a salad in place of fries, pasta, or other starchy sides is so common today that it's not even really a special request.

The one problem place is a pizza restaurant. There's nothing quite like a slice or two of pizza to send your blood sugar rocketing upward. You eat most of the toppings—ask them to hold the sauces and don't eat the crust.

Eat pizza only if you're trapped on a desert island or it's the only food between you and starvation. Does this mean you'll have to bring your lunch or find something else to eat on pizza Friday at work? Yes. You're a grown-up—you'll figure it out.

When Traveling

- Plan ahead—know when and where your major pitfalls will come, so that you can plan to avoid them. If you're going to eat healthy while traveling, you must prepare yourself and make your diet a priority.
- Follow the 80/20 rule—when traveling, it's difficult to be 100 percent perfect. Aim to eat healthy 80 percent of the time. A missed meal or poor snack choice every now and then is to be expected. Just make sure it's the exception to the rule.
- Bring the basics with you—high-quality jerky, fruits, sliced veggies (like celery, carrots, broccoli), nuts, and seeds. A few great prepackaged sources for healthy snacks are found at awesomefoods.com (they sell raw, vegan snacks, including cashew and pistachio nut sticks; vegetable chips like kale, carrot, beet, yam, and onion; and vegan crackers made with veggies, soaked nuts, and seeds) or stevesoriginal.com (they sell great paleokits that include grass-fed jerky, dried fruit, nuts in a vacuum-sealed pack—perfect for traveling).

- Choose hotels wisely—try to pick hotels with a fridge and mini-kitchen. If that's not possible, then request a mini-fridge in your hotel room in advance.
- If you weren't able to pack some of your own snacks before you left, once you've arrived at your destination, go to the closest grocery and buy some organic, sliced veggies, a few apples, 3 or 4 ounces of nuts, a few avocados, and slices of nitrate-free sliced meats like Applegate Farms brand.
- Frequent hotels catering to business travelers and take advantage of complimentary healthful foods—hard-boiled or scrambled eggs, bacon, fruit, nuts, etc. Hotel lounge areas may have a supply of fruits and nuts readily available. Skip the complimentary cookies.
- If you're driving to your destination, bring a cooler and stock up on the aforementioned foods. For longer road trips, periodically make "pit stops" at grocery stores and restock.
- Some "lesser evil" fast-food choices can be found—burgers without the bun or wrapped in lettuce leaves; do the same with Subway sandwiches. At Chipotle, for example, order the "burrito bowl." Most fast-food restaurants have salads—just add some chicken or steak and avocado slices to make it more satisfying. However, beware of the salad dressings, which are usually loaded with sugars. Just ask for olive oil and vinegar on the side.

In Restaurants

Don't be afraid to be picky when ordering your meals at restaurants. Order fish, chicken, or meat grilled and plain; ask for steamed vegetables instead of fries or baked potatoes; get sauces on the side.

- **Breakfast food:** Find a little diner and order bacon and eggs or an omelet with your favorite veggies.

- **Mexican food:** Choose fajitas and skip the tortillas.

- **Steak house:** Eat a steak with veggies and/or salad. Skip the potatoes.

- **Sushi:** Avoid the rice and order the sashimi, or simply avoid any entrée that contains mostly rice.

- **Seafood:** All choices of seafood would be acceptable, but choose dishes with no breading. Order with a side salad and/or veggies.

- **American food:** Avoid buns, bread, fries, and chips—no breading on anything! Ask to have your burger plain or choose baked fish, poultry, or eggs.

- **Italian food:** Watch for carbohydrate overload here—just ask for fresh fish or chicken breast with butter or olive oil (no breading), or plain meat. A good alternative is to order a large antipasto salad.

Let's recap.

1. Eating a low-carbohydrate diet high in grass-fed animal fat and protein will reduce blood sugar and insulin levels.
2. Good fats increase HDL levels and lower blood triglycerides.
3. Removing sugar from your diet will radically halt the inflammation of all the nerves within your body, reduce damage, and stop the pain of peripheral neuropathy.

Unbeknownst to the general public, we have all been put into a chemical state of gluttony by the hidden sugars in our food. When unchecked, this can keep you in a constant cycle of hunger and bingeing. Instead, this book shows you how to enjoy the state of true satiation. Doing so will transform your life. Just put healthy fat in your diet. Then you will no longer be a slave to food.

Sugar is the problem and fat is the answer.

Epilogue

MY OWN AWAKENING

I was fifty years old and more than twenty years into my medical career when an emergency gallbladder removal forced me to reevaluate my beliefs about what constituted a healthy lifestyle.

I'd always gotten plenty of exercise and followed the recommendations in the USDA food pyramid. No one ever guessed my age. My basic diet and exercise patterns were consistently on target and I felt great—right up to the moment I was doubled over by the agonizing pain of a gallbladder attack. If you've never experienced this (and I hope you haven't, and never will), let me just say that, in the emergency room, gallbladder attacks are often mistaken for heart attacks—and vice versa.

When I asked the ER doctor what had happened, all she could say was that some people have an inherited tendency toward gallbladder problems. That made some sense to me at the time, because my mother's gallbladder was removed when she was about my age. Even so, I had questions the doctor couldn't answer. Even among people with a genetic tendency toward gallbladder stones, why do only some of us actually get them? Why do gallbladder issues seem to show up in middle age? And does diet have anything to do with it?

All the surgeon seemed to say was, "We got that gallbladder out with no problem. Relax. Forget about it; you're fine."

Shortly thereafter, I ran into my family doctor in the lunchroom of the hospital. He asked how I was doing and I told him about the surgery.

"Well," he said, "you're not exercising it; after all, the gallbladder is a muscle. You need to eat more."

Mind you, he was obese.

Okay, I thought, he could be right—if it's a muscle, it needs to be exercised. I rarely ate breakfast and my hospital lunches were hit-or-miss, and full of carbs. Full dinners often included late-night overeating. I decided right there to discover all I could about my disease and figure out what I could do to improve my health.

The mission of this book has been to encourage you to do the same.

What Will It Take for You to Change?

In some states cigarette cartons have photos of diseased lungs meant to jar you into a positive action—to stop smoking. I could show you pictures of surgical procedures that could freak you out; but after reading this book, I hope that's not necessary.

Consider the alternatives; and if there's only a small chance I'm correct, and if all you have to do is cut out sugar— why not give it a try?

No need to fret over diet plans or fear you'll never overcome a lifetime of bad habits. Change can be difficult at first, but recognize that you're not alone. You and everyone else in America has been educated into ignorance—about sugar and fat, about bread and pasta, about artificial sweeteners, about high-fructose corn syrup, and about the bucolic loveliness of soy. You've paid for this education with your tax dollars and your health.

The nerve of it! This colossal cover-up literally dwarfs the tobacco story.

After reading this book, you need only remember a few fundamental concepts:

- Stop eating sugar.
- Start eating good animal fats (from grass-fed sources).
- And don't steal honey from the bees. It feeds new, baby bees and we need them to help pollinate the planet.

Taking control of your diet will do more to keep you healthy than an endless array of drugs designed to fill the pockets of robber barons. And just because you have a genetic predisposition for a disease does not make it inevitable that you'll contract that illness.

Remember, the traditional nomenclature of medicine does not look at cause; it looks at effect. We need to step back from the old paradigm and view disease through the lens of global nerve compression.

It's a simple, causal formulation:

Sugar + Refined Carbohydrates =
Inflammation + Trauma = Nerve Damage

ACKNOWLEDGMENTS

————

Joint Acknowledgments

Our deepest appreciation goes out to Al Zuckerman, one of the most famous and successful literary agents in the world, having worked with authors like Stephen Hawking and his book *A Brief History of Time*, Ken Follett, and numerous other successful writers. The first time we spoke he referred to our work as "a profound and revolutionary book." We were humbled and grateful. We also want to thank Karen Rinaldi, our publisher at Harper Wave, for her encouragement and vision for the book.

Thank you to Madison Turbeville for all of her great organization, research, and development of source materials for the book; Annette Lyon, office manager; Lisa Heard, laboratory assistant, and the rest of the staff of Valley Foot Surgeons, who were invaluable contributors to this manuscript; Sheila Buff for all she did to help us build the manuscript; and Jill Bernstein, our incredible editor. Jill, your brilliant work helped elevate this book to a whole new level.

Personal Acknowledgments

Dr. Jacoby

Without a phenomenal cast of writers and contributors, this book would not have been possible. Obviously there are too many in the cast to give credit to all, but the single most important person in this book obviously is Lee Dellon, M.D., Ph.D. Without Lee's insight and perseverance and his work at Johns Hopkins and his friendship, this book would not have been possible. People like John Cooke, M.D., Ph.D., from Stanford, who was an early adopter of my ideas, Michael Hamblin, Ph.D., from Harvard, Martin Pall, Ph.D., from Washington State University, Aaron Filler, M.D., Ph.D., from the University of California, Los Angeles, and Melvin Hayden, M.D., who all accepted my invitation to come to the Association of Extremity Nerve Surgeons to explain their science to our group. Additionally, Bob Parker, D.P.M., was invaluable in encouraging me to write down my thoughts, as was the friendship of Brian McDowell, D.P.M. Thank you to Fred Marciano, M.D., Ph.D., neurosurgeon, who was invaluable in encouraging me to pursue the Dellon approach; Steve Barrett, D.P.M., who introduced Dellon concepts into podiatry; and Gene Livingston, D.P.M., for his research on the subject.

Early on in this process, I traveled to New York to meet with Al and have dinner with him and his wife, Claire, at their lovely home in Manhattan. He is a very gracious and interesting man, and we talked of many things. At one point he mentioned having seen the play *Bullets Over Broadway*, and, even though it got mixed reviews, said how much he enjoyed it. The next night I saw the play and I also thought it was excellent. It resonated with what I have tried to accomplish in this book. First, it has a lot to say about maintaining a commitment to your ideals. Second, it shows that the world looks very different, depending on your perspective. If you look at something from the expected viewpoint, you're going to see what's expected. But if you step back and look at it from a different angle, with fresh eyes, you can see old problems in an entirely new way. In many ways, this book is my "Bullets Over Medicine."

I would finally like to thank my coauthor, Raquel Baldelomar. Her persistence in keeping the project moving over the last two years was invaluable.

Raquel

There are several people whom I would like to thank for helping me with this book and being such a strong influence in my life. I would like to thank my mother, Susan, who taught me that instinct won't carry us through this entire journey. It's what we do in the moments between inspiration that will define our success. I also want to thank my cousin, Katie Gilbert, who guided me to the right people to get this book off the ground. I want to thank Jerry Short for believing in me and pushing me to own my life, not rent it. You gave me the tools necessary to help me build a thriving business, and I will forever be grateful for your wisdom and guidance. I want to thank the many clients that have become almost like family to me. You took a chance on me and our small ad agency, particularly Dr. Monte Swarup. I want to thank my entire staff and close friends for helping me maintain conscious attention to the things that matter most, particularly Matthew Dinnerman, Omar Faruk, Kathleen Rachael, Sarah Hollander, Marc Finer, Matt Lane, Connie Zweig,

Reza Iranpour, and Michael Chernis. My biggest thanks go to Dr. Jacoby for being on this journey with me these last seven years and trusting me to write this book with you. You taught me the necessity of persistence and that nothing good is ever easy.

BIBLIOGRAPHY

1: THE 500-POUND CANARY

"Antioxidants: Beyond the Hype." *Nutrition Source.* www.hsph.harvard .edu/nutritionsource/antioxidants.

Challem, Jack. *The Inflammation Syndrome.* Hoboken, NJ: John Wiley, 2003.

Dufault, R., B. LeBlanc, R. Schnoll, et al. "Mercury from Chlor-Alkali Plants: Measured Concentrations in Product Sugar." *Environmental Health*, 2009.

Lustig, Robert H. "Sugar: The Bitter Truth." University of California, San Francisco, video. www.youtube.com/watch?v=dBnniua6-oM.

University of California Television. www.uctv.tv/sugar-the-bitter-truth-167.

Wallinga, David, M.D., Janelle Sorensen, Pooja Mottl, and Brian Yablon, M.D. "Not So Sweet: Missing Mercury and High Fructose Corn Syrup." Institute for Agriculture and Trade Policy, Minneapolis, Minnesota, 2009.

Web Medicine. www.webmed.com/food-recipies/features/how-antioxidants-work1.

Willett, Walter. *Eat, Drink and Be Healthy.* New York: Free Press, 2005.

Yang, Q., et al. "Added Sugar Intake and Cardiovascular Diseases Mortality among US Adults." *JAMA Internal Medicine* 174, no. 4 (April 2014): 516–24.

Yudkin, John, and Robert H. Lustig. *Pure, White, and Deadly: How Sugar Is Killing Us and What We Can Do to Stop It*. New York: Penguin, 2013.

2: THE NERVE OF IT ALL

Bryan, Nathan S. "Nitric Oxide and Diabetes: The Deadly Cardiovascular Implications of Insulin Resistance." www.integrativepractioner.com/article.aspx?id=19330.

Ducker, T. B. "Pathophysiology of Peripheral Nerve Trauma." In G. E. Omar, ed., *Management of Peripheral Nerve Problems*. Philadelphia: W. B. Saunders, 1980, p. 476.

Guyuron, B., et al. "Five-Year Outcome of Surgical Treatment of Migraine Headaches." *Plastic Reconstructive Surgery* 127, no. 2 (February 2011): 603–8.

Perkins, Bruce A., et al. "Carpal Tunnel Syndrome in Patients with Diabetic Polyneuropathy." *Diabetes Care* 25, no. 3 (March 2002): 565–69.

Schulman, S. P., L. C. Becker, D. A. Kass, et al. "L-Arginine Therapy in Acute Myocardial Infarction: The Vascular Interaction with Age in Myocardial Infarction (VINTAGE MI) Randomized Clinical Trial." *JAMA* 295, no. 1 (January 2006): 58–64.

3: KILLING YOU SOFTLY

Aszmann, O. C., K. M. Kress, and A. Dellon. "Results of Decompression of Peripheral Nerves in Diabetics: A Prospective, Blinded Study." *Plastic Reconstructive Surgery* 106, no. 4 (September 2000): 816–22.

Boden, G., H. Sargrad, C. Homko, M. Mozzoli, and T. P. Stein. "Effect of a Low-Carbohydrate Diet on Appetite, Blood Glucose Levels, and Insulin Resistance in Obese Patients with Type 2 Diabetes." *Annals of Internal Medicine* 142, no. 6 (March 2005): 403–11.

Chaudhry, V., J. Stevens, J. Kincaid, and Y. So. "Practice Advisory: Utility of Surgical Decompression for Treatment of Diabetic Neuropathy: Report of the Therapeutics and Technology Assessment Subcommittee of the American Academy of Neurology." *Neurology* 66, no. 12 (2006): 1805–08.

Cooke, John. "Asymmetrical Dimethylargine: The Uber Marker?" *Circulation*, 2004.

Cornblath, D. R., et al. "Surgical Decompression for Diabetic Senso-rimotor Polyneuropathy." *Diabetes Care* 30, no. 2 (February 2007): 421–22.

Dellon, A. L. "Treatment of Symptomatic Diabetic Neuropathy by Surgical Decompression of Multiple Peripheral Nerves." *Plastic Reconstructive Surgery* 89, no. 4 (April 1992): 698–99.

Dellon, A. L., V. L. Muse, D. S. Nickerson, et al. "Prevention of Ulceration, Amputation, and Reduction of Hospitalization: Outcomes of a Prospective Multicenter Trial of Tibial Neurolysis in Patients with Diabetic Neuropathy." *Journal of Reconstructive Microsurgery* 28, no. 4 (2012): 241–46.

"Diabetic Neuropathy: A Small-Fiber Disease." *Medscape Multispecialty*, www.medscape.org/viewarticle/418568.

Groner, C. "Nerve Decompression and Diabetic Neuropathy." *Lower Extremity Review*, January 2014.

Lee, C., and A. L. Dellon. "Prognostic Ability of Tinel Sign in Determining Outcome for Decompression Surgery in Diabetic and Non-Diabetic Neuropathy." *Annals of Plastic Surgery* 53 (2004): 523–27.

Nickerson, D. S., and A. J. Rader. "Low Long-Term Risk of Foot Ulcer Recurrence After Nerve Decompression in a Diabetes Neuropathy Cohort." *Journal of the American Podiatric Medicine Association.* 103, no. 5 (September–October 2013): 380–86.

Malik, V. S., et al. "Sugar-Sweetened Beverages and Risk of Metabolic Syndrome and Type 2 Diabetes: A Meta-Analysis." *Diabetes Care* 33, no. 11 (November 2010): 2477–83.

Pecket, P., and A. Schattner. "Concurrent Bell's Palsy and Diabetes Mellitus: A Diabetic Mononeuropathy?" *Journal of Neurology Neurosurgery and Psychiatry* 45, no. 7 (July 1982): 652–55.

Rydevik, B. L. "The Effects of Compression on the Physiology of Nerve Roots." *Journal of Manipulative Physiological Therapeutics* 15, no. 1 (January 1992): 62–66.

Seyfried, Thomas. *Cancer as a Metabolic Disease: On the Origin, Management, and Prevention of Cancer.* New York: Wiley, 2012.

Siemionow, M., M. Alghoul, M. Molski, and G. Agaoglu. "Clinical Outcome of Peripheral Nerve Decompression in Diabetic and Non-Diabetic Peripheral Neuropathy." *Annals of Plastic Surgery* 57, no. 4 (2006): 385–90.

Therapeutics and Technology Assessment Subcommittee of the American Academy of Neurology, V. Chaudhry, J. C. Stevens, J. Kincaid, and Y. T. So. "Practice Advisory: Utility of Surgical Decompression for Treatment of Diabetic Neuropathy." Report of the Therapeutics and Technology Assessment Subcommittee of the American Academy of Neurology. *Neurology* 66, no. 12 (June 2006): 1805–08.

Thony, B., et al. "Tetrahydrobiopterin Biosynthesis, Regeneration, and Functions." *Biochemical Journal* 374, no.1 (April 1, 2000):1–16.

Tseng, C. L., et al. "Assessing Potential Glycemic Overtreatment in Persons at Hypoglycemic Risk." *JAMA Internal Medicine* 174, no. 2 (February 2014): 259–68.

Tucker, Miriam E. "Nerve Decompression Debate Continues in Diabetic Neuropathy." *Medscape*, February 17, 2014. www.medscape.com/viewarticle/820691.

Upton, A. R., and A. J. McComas. "The Double Crush in Nerve Entrapment Syndromes." *Lancet* 2, no. 7825 (August 18, 1973): 359–62.

Valdivia, J. M. V., et al. "Surgical Treatment of Peripheral Neuropathy: Outcomes from 100 Consecutive Decompressions." *Journal of American Podiatric Medical Association* 95 (2005): 451–54.

Wieman, T. J., and V. G. Patel. "Treatment of Hyperesthetic Neuropathic Pain in Diabetics: Decompression of the Tarsal Tunnel." *Annals of Surgery* 22, no. 6 (June 1995): 660–64; discussion 664–65.

Yang, Quanhe, Ph.D., et al. "Added Sugar Intake and Cardiovascular Diseases Mortality among US Adults." *JAMA Internal Medicine* 174, no. 4 (2014): 516–24.

4: SLIGHTLY DIABETIC

Addolorato, G., et al. "Regional Cerebral Hypoperfusion in Patients with Celiac Disease." *American Journal of Medicine* 116, no. 5 (March 2004): 312–17.

American Diabetes Association. www.diabetes.org/are-you-at-risk/prediabetes/.

ALS Association. www.alsa.org/news/archive/nfl-players-risk.html.

Burke, L. M., et al. "Guidelines for Daily Carbohydrate Intake: Do Athletes Achieve Them?" *Sports Medicine* 31, no. 4 (2001): 267–99.

Choudhry, Oshamah, et al. "Historical Evolution of the Microvascular

Decompression Procedure for Trigeminal Neuroglia: From Dandy to Jannetta." *World Science*, 2012, www.world-sci.com/read.aspx?id=871.

de la Monte, Suzanne. "Alzheimer's: Diabetes of the Brain?" Alpert Medical School, Brown University, electronic posting, April 6, 2011.

Dellon, A. L. "Susceptibility of Nerve in Diabetes to Compression: Implications for Pain Treatment." *Plastic and Reconstructive Surgery* 134, no. 4S-2 (October 2014: 142S–150S.

Ford, R. P. "The Gluten Syndrome: A Neurological Disease." *Medical Hypotheses* 73, no. 3 (September 2009): 438–40.

Giovannucci, E., et al. "Diabetes and Cancer: A Consensus Report." *Diabetes Care* 33, no. 7 (July 2010): 1674–85.

"The Gluten Syndrome: A Neurological Disease." www.mayoclinic.org diseases-conditions/diabetes/in-depth/blood-sugar/.

Gray, Henry. *Anatomy, Descriptive and Surgical*. Classic Edition. Philadelphia: Running Press, 1974.

Hassaidou, Maria. "Carbohydrate Requirements of Elite Athletes." *British Journal of Sports Medicine*, 2011;45e2 doi:10,1136.

Hu, W. T., et al. "Cognitive Impairment and Celiac Disease." *Archives of Neurology* 63, no. 10 (October 2006): 1440–46.

Hubbard Foundation. www.hubbardfoundation.org.

Isomaa, B., et al. "Cardiovascular Morbidity and Mortality Associated with the Metabolic Syndrome." *Diabetes Care* 24, no. 4 (April 2001): 683–89.

"The Link between Diabetes and Cancer . . . and Reducing the Risk of Both." American Institute for Cancer Research, Health@Work, November 11, 2013.

Markram, H., T. Rinaldi, and K. Markram. "The Intense World Syndrome: An Alternative Hypothesis for Autism." *Frontiers in Neuroscience* 1, no. 1 (October 2007): 77–96.

Ohara, T., et al. "Glucose Tolerance Status and Risk of Dementia in the Community: The Hisayama Study." *Neurology* 77, no. 12 (September 2011): 1126–34.

Pall, Martin L. *Explaining "Unexplained Illnesses": Disease Paradigm for Chronic Fatigue Syndrome, Multiple Chemical Sensitivity, Fibromyalgia, Post-Traumatic Stress Disorder, and Gulf War Syndrome*. London: CRC Press, 2007.

Perry, G., et al. "Oxidative Damage in the Olfactory System in Alzheimer's Disease." *Acta Neuropathologica* 106, no. 6 (2003): 562–66.

Pinto, Jayant M., et al. "Olfactory Dysfunction Predicts 5-year Mortality in Older Adults." *PLOS-One*, October 1, 2014. DCI:10,1371/journal .pone.0107541.

Rodier, Patricia M. "The Early Origins of Autism." *Scientific American*, February 2000, pp. 56–63.

Rodier, P. M., et al. "Embryological Origin for Autism: Developmental Anomalies of the Cranial Nerve Motor Nuclei." *Journal of Comparative Neurology* 370, no. 2 (June 1996): 247–61.

Seyfried, Thomas N., Roberto Flores, Angela M. Poff, and Dominic P. D'Agostino. "Cancer as a Metabolic Disease: Implications for Novel Therapeutics." *Carcinogenesis* 35, no. 3 (March 2014): 515–27.

"Spotlight on the Gut Bacteria-Brain Connection in Autism," November 13, 2013, www.autismspeaks.org/science/science-news.

"The Suicide Disease-Trigeminal Neuralgia or Tic Douloureux." www.medfaxxinc.com/index.php?/Articles/the-suicide-disease-trigeminal-neuralgia-or-tic-douloureux.html.

Taubes, Gary. "Is Sugar Toxic?" *New York Times Magazine*, April 17, 2011, p. MM47.

Tseng, C. H. "Benign Prostatic Hyperplasia Is a Significant Risk Factor for Bladder Cancer in Diabetic Patients: A Population-Based Cohort Study Using the National Health Insurance in Taiwan." *BMC Cancer* 13 (January 2013): 7.

Tullis, Paul. "A Controversial 'Cure' for M.S." *New York Times Magazine*, October 26, 2012.

Wahls, T. L. "The Seventy Percent Solution." *Journal of General Internal Medicine* 26, no. 10 (October 2011): 1215–16.

Wang, Shirley. "Key to Detecting Alzheimer's Early Could Be in the Eye." *Wall Street Journal*, July 14, 2014.

Yang, Q., et al. "Added Sugar Intake and Cardiovascular Diseases Mortality among US Adults." *JAMA Internal Medicine* 174, no. 4 (April 2014): 516–24.

Zimmer, Carl. *Soul Made Flesh: The Discovery of the Brain—and How It Changed the World*. New York: Atria Books, 2005.

5: ON TRACK FOR NERVE DAMAGE

Callaghan, B. C., et al. "Triglycerides and Amputation Risk in Patients with Diabetes: Ten-Year Follow-Up in the DISTANCE Study." *Diabetes Care* 34, no. 3 (March 2011): 635–40.

"Carpal Tunnel Syndrome." American Accreditation Healthcare Commission, September 30, 2014, University of Maryland Medical Center, October 2014, http://umm.edu/health/medical/altmed/condition/carpal-tunnel-syndrome.

Choudhry, O., et al. "Historical Evolution of the Microvascular Decompression Theory for Trigeminal Neuralgia: From Dandy to Jannetta." *World Science*, 2012, www.world-sci.com/read.aspx?id=871.

Danby, F. W. "Nutrition and Acne." *Clinical Dermatology* 28, no. 6 (November–December 2010): 598–604.

Gill, J. M., and N. Sattar. "Fruit Juice: Just Another Sugary Drink?" *Lancet Diabetes & Endocrinology* 2, no. 6 (June 2014): 444–46.

Groner, C. "Nerve Decompression and Diabetic Neuropathy." *Lower Extremity Review*, January 2014.

Gruber, H. J., et al. "Hyperinsulinaemia in Migraineurs Is Associated with Nitric Oxide Stress." *Cephalalgia* 30, no. 5 (May 2010): 593–98.

Guyuron, B., J. S. Kriegler, J. Davis, and S. B. Amini. "Comprehensive Surgical Treatment of Migraine Headaches." *Plastic Reconstructive Surgery* 115, no. 1 (January 2005): 1–9.

Hang, Yuli. "Screen for Prediabetes Using ADA Criteria for Cancer Prevention." *Diabetologia*, September 8, 2014, www.diabetologia-journal.org.

Hitti, Miranda. "Carpal Tunnel May Predict Diabetes." *WebMD Health News*, www.webmd.com.

"Men and Migraine." www.themigrainetrust.org.

Merlino, G., et al. "Association of Restless Legs Syndrome in Type 2 Diabetes: A Case-Control Study." *Sleep* 30, no. 7 (July 2007): 866–71.

Pfeffer, G. B., et al. "The History of Carpal Tunnel Syndrome." *Journal of Hand Surgery: British* 13, no. 1 (February 1988): 28–34.

Smith, R. N., et al. "A Low-Glycemic-Load Diet Improves Symptoms in Acne Vulgaris Patients: A Randomized Controlled Trial." *American Journal of Clinical Nutrition* 86, no. 1 (July 2007): 107–15.

Strauss, S. M., et al. "The Dental Office Visit as a Potential Opportunity for Diabetes Screening: An Analysis Using NHANES 2003–2004 Data." *Journal of Public Health Dentistry* 70, no. 2 (Spring 2010): 156–62.

Wiggin, T. D., et al. "Elevated Triglycerides Correlate with Progression of Diabetic Neuropathy." *Diabetes* 58, no. 7 (July 2009): 1634–40.

Zakrzewska, J. M., and H. Akram. "Neurosurgical Interventions for the Treatment of Classical Trigeminal Neuralgia." Cochrane Database of Systematic Reviews, September 7, 2011, CD007312.

6: THE FIVE PHASES OF PERIPHERAL NEUROPATHY

"Alcoholic Neuropathy." MedlinePlus, U.S. National Library of Medicine, National Institutes of Health, www.nim.nih.gov/medlineplus/ency/article/000714.htm.

7: MEANWHILE, JUST MAKE IT STOP

Ang, C. D., et al. "Vitamin B for Treating Peripheral Neuropathy." *Cochrane Database of Systematic Reviews* 16 (July 2008): CD004573.

Brownrigg, J. R., et al. "The Association of Ulceration of the Foot with Cardiovascular and All-Cause Mortality in Patients with Diabetes: A Meta-Analysis." *Diabetologia* 55, no. 11 (November 2012): 2906–12.

Bryhn, M., H. Hansteen, T. Schanche, and S. E. Aakre. "Prostaglandins, Leukotrienes and Essential Fatty Acids: The Bioavailability and Pharmacodynamics of Different Concentrations of Omega-3 Acid Ethyl Esters." *Science Direct* 75, no. 1 (July 2006): 19–24.

Dibaba, D. T., et. al, "Dietary Magnesium Intake's Role in Decreasing Metabolic Syndrome." *Diabetic Medicine*, November, 2014.

Dworkin, Robert H., Ph.D., et al. "Recommendations for the Pharmacological Management of Neuropathic Pain: An Overview and Literature Update." *Mayo Clinic Proceedings* 85, 3 Suppl. (March 2010): S3–S14.

Forouhi, N. G., et al. "Baseline Serum 25-Hydroxy Vitamin D Is Predictive of Future Glycemic Status and Insulin resistance: The Medical Research Council Ely Prospective Study 1990-2000." *Diabetes* 57 (2008): 2619–25.

Fossel, E. T. "Improvement of Temperature and Flow in Feet of Subjects with Diabetes with Use of a Transdermal Preparation of L-Arginine: A Pilot Study." *Diabetes Care* 27, no. 1 (January 2004): 284–85.

Gaist, D., et al. "Statins and Risk of Polyneuropathy: A Case-Control Study." *Neurology* 58, no. 0 (May 2002): 1333–37.

Halat, K. M., and C. E. Dennehy. "Botanicals and Dietary Supplements in Diabetic Peripheral Neuropathy. *Journal of the American Board of Family Practice* 16, no. 1 (2003): 47–57.

Hruby, Adela, et al. "Higher Magnesium Intake Reduces Risk of Impaired Glucose and Insulin Metabolism, and Progression from Prediabetes to Diabetes in Middle-Aged Americans." *Diabetes Care* 37, no. 2 (February 2014): 419–27.

Kao, W. H., et al. "Serum and Dietary Magnesium and the Risk for Type 2 Diabetes Mellitus: The Atherosclerosis Risk in Communities Study." *Archives of Internal Medicine* 159, no. 18 (October 1999): 2151–59.

Keen, H., J. Payan, J. Allawi, et al. "Treatment of Diabetic Neuropathy with Gamma-Linolenic Acid. The Gamma-Linolenic Acid Multicenter Trial Group." *Diabetes Care* 16, no. 1 (1993): 8–15.

Larsson, S. C., and A. Wolk. "Magnesium Intake and Risk of Type 2 Diabetes: A Meta-Analysis." *Journal of Internal Medicine* 262, no. 2 (August 2007): 208–14.

Low, P. A., et al. "Double-Blind, Placebo-Controlled Study of the Application of Capsaicin Cream in Chronic Distal Painful Polyneuropathy." *Pain* 62, no. 2 (1995): 163–68.

McNicol, E. D., A. Midbari, and E. Eisenberg. "Opioids for Neuropathic Pain." *Cochrane Database of Systematic Reviews*, August 29, 2013.

Norhammar, A., et al. "Glucose Metabolism in Patients with Acute Myocardial Infarction and No Previous Diagnosis of Diabetes Mellitus: A Prospective Study." *Lancet* 359, no. 9324 (June 2002): 2140–44.

Odell, Robert H., Jr. "New Device Combines Electrical Currents and Local Anesthetic for Pain Management." *Practical Pain Management* 11, no. 6 (2011): 52–68.

Possidente, C. J., and R. Tandan. "A Survey of Treatment Practices in Diabetic Peripheral Neuropathy." *Primary Care Diabetes* 3, no. 4 (November 2009): 253–57.

Ridker, Paul M., et al. "Cardiovascular Benefits and Diabetes Risks of Statin Therapy in Primary Prevention: An Analysis from the JUPITER Trial." *Lancet* 380, no. 9841 (August 2012): 565–71.

Rodríguez-Morán, M., and F. Guerrero-Romero. "Low Serum Magnesium Levels and Foot Ulcers in Subjects with Type 2 Diabetes." *Archives of Medical Research* 32, no. 4 (July–August 2001): 300–303.

Sugiyama, Takehiro, et al. "Different Time Trends of Caloric and Fat Intake Between Statin Users and Nonusers Among US Adults: Gluttony in the Time of Statins?" *JAMA Internal Medicine*, online, April 24, 2014, doi:10.1001/jamainternmed.2014.

Tandan, R., et al. "Topical Capsaicin in Painful Diabetic Neuropathy: Controlled Study with Long-Term Follow-Up." *Diabetes Care* 15, no. 1 (1992): 8–14.

Wiffen, P. J., S. Derry, M. P. Lunn, and R. A. Moore. "Topiramate for Neuropathic Pain and Fibromyalgia in Adults." *Cochrane Database of Systematic Reviews*, August 30, 2013.

Wong, Man-chun, Joanne W. Y. Chung, and Thomas K. S. Wong. "Effects of Treatments for Symptoms of Painful Diabetic Neuropathy: Systematic Review." *British Medical Journal* 335, no. 7610 (July 2007): 87.

Yamanya, Abeer A., and Hayam M. Sayed. "Effect of Low Level Laser Therapy on Neurovascular Function of Diabetic Peripheral Neuropathy." *Journal of Advanced Research* 3, no. 1 (January 2012): 21–28.

Zang, Kerry, et al. "Can Low-Level Laser Therapy Have an Impact for Small Fiber Neuropathy?" *Podiatry Today* 24, no. 6 (June 2011).

Ziegler, D., et al. "Efficacy and Safety of Antioxidant Treatment with á-Lipoic Acid over 4 Years in Diabetic Polyneuropathy: The NATHAN 1 Trial." *Diabetes Care* 34, no. 9 (September 2011): 2054–60.

Ziegler, D., et al. "Oral Treatment with Alpha-Lipoic Acid Improves Symptomatic Diabetic Polyneuropathy: The SYDNEY 2 Trial." *Diabetes Care* 29, no. 11 (November 2006): 2365–70.

Zinman, Lorne H., et al. "Low-Intensity Laser Therapy for Painful Symptoms of Diabetic Sensorimotor Polyneuropathy: A Controlled Trial." *Diabetes Care* 27, no. 4 (April 2004): 921–24.

8: THE SUGAR ADDICTION

Ascherio, A., et al. "Dietary Fat and Risk of Coronary Heart Disease in Men: Cohort Follow-Up Study in the United States." *British Medical Journal* 313, no. 7049 (July 1996): 84–90.

Beauchamp, G. K., and P. Pearson. "Human Development and Umami Taste." *Physiology & Behavior* 49, no. 5 (1991): 1009–12.

Benton, D. "Carbohydrate Ingestion, Blood Glucose, and Mood." *Neuroscience Biobehavioral Reviews* 26, no. 3 (May 2002): 293–308.

Cernak, Cynthia, et al. "Combination Electrochemical Therapy (CET) to Treat Patients with Diabetic Neuropathy." *Regional Anesthesia and Pain Medicine* 35, no. 5 (September/October 2010): 459–70.

Greer, Stephanie, Andrea N. Goldstein, and Matthew P. Walker. "The Impact of Sleep Deprivation on Food Desire in the Human Brain." *Nature Communications* 4, no. 2259, August 6, 2013.

Kam, Katherine. "The Facts on Leptin: FAQ, the Truth About the Hormone Leptin and Obesity." WebMD Archive, March 11, 2010, www.webmd.com/diet/features/the-facts-on-lepin-faq?page=2.

Keckeis, Marietta, et al. "Impaired Glucose Tolerance in Sleep Disorders." *PLoS One* 5, no. 3 (2010): e9444.

Lennerz, Belinda S., et al. "Effects of Dietary Glycemic Index on Brain Regions Related to Reward and Craving in Men." *American Journal of Clinical Nutrition*, September 2013.

Lenoir, Magalie, Fuschia Serre, et al. "Intense Sweetness Surpasses Cocaine Reward." *PLOS One*, August 1, 2007, doi:10:1371/journal.pone.0000698.

Peters, John C., et al. "The Effects of Water and Non-Nutritive Sweetened Beverages on Weight Loss During a 12-Week Weight Loss Treatment Program." *Obesity*, May 26, 2014, doi:10.1002/oby.20737.

Polyzos, S. A., et al. "The Potential Adverse Role of Leptin Resistance in Nonalcoholic Fatty Liver Disease: A Hypothesis Based on Critical Review of the Literature." *Journal of Clinical Gastroenterology* 45, no. 1 (January 2011): 50–54.

U.S. Air Force. "Aspartame Alert." *Flying Safely*, May 1992, pp. 20–21.

9: THE BIG FAT LIE

Beglinger, Christoph, and Lukas Degen. "Fat in the Intestine as a Regulator of Appetite: Role of CCK." *Physiology & Behavior* 83 (2004): 617–21.

Boden, G., et al. "Effect of a Low-Carbohydrate Diet on Appetite, Blood Glucose Levels, and Insulin Resistance in Obese Patients with Type 2 Diabetes." *Annals of Internal Medicine* 142, no. 6 (March 2005): 403–11.

Chowdhury, Rajiv, et al. "Association of Dietary, Circulating, and Supplement Fatty Acids with Coronary Risk." *Annals of Internal Medicine* 160, no. 6 (March 2014): 398–406.

Geary, N. "Estradiol, CCK, and Satiation." *Peptides* 22, no. 8 (August 2001): 1251–63.

Gill, J. M., and N. Sattar. "Fruit Juice: Just Another Sugary Drink?" *Lancet Diabetes & Endocrinology* 2, no. 6 (June 2014): 444–46.

Kasarda, D. D. "Can an Increase in Celiac Disease Be Attributed to an Increase in the Gluten Content of Wheat as a Consequence of Wheat Breeding?" *Journal of Agriculture and Food Chemistry* 61, no. 6 (2013): 1155–59.

Krebs-Smith, Susan M., Jill Reedy, and Claire Bosire. "Healthfulness of the U.S. Food Supply: Little Improvement Despite Decades of Dietary Guidance." *American Journal of Preventative Medicine* 38, no. 5 (May 2010): 472–77.

Kris-Etherton, Penny, et al., for the Nutrition Committee Population Science Committee and Clinical Science Committee of the American Heart Association. AHA Science Advisory. Lyon Diet Heart Study. "Benefits of a Mediterranean-Style, National Cholesterol Education Program/American Heart Association Step I Dietary Pattern on Cardiovascular Disease." *Circulation* 103 (2001): 1823–25.

"Managing Your Cholesterol." With Mason Freeman, M.D., chief of the Lipid Metabolism Unit, Massachusetts General Hospital. *Harvard Health Publications*, 2014, www.health.harvard.edu.

Mozaffarian, D., et al. "Trans Fatty Acids and Cardiovascular Disease." *New England Journal of Medicine* 354 (2006): 1601–13.

Nestle, Marion. *Food Politics: How the Food Industry Influences Nutrition and Health.* Berkeley: University of California Press, 2002.

Rumawas, M. E., et al. "Magnesium Intake Is Related to Improved In-
    sulin Homeostasis in the Framingham Offspring Cohort." *Journal
    of the American College of Nutrition* 25, no. 6 (December 2006):
    486–92.

Salas-Salvadó, J., et al. "Prevention of Diabetes with Mediterranean
    Diets: A Subgroup Analysis of a Randomized Trial." *Annals of Inter-
    nal Medicine* 160, no. 1 (January 2014): 1–10.

Siri-Tarino, Patty B., et al. "Meta-analysis of Prospective Cohort Studies
    Evaluating the Association of Saturated Fat with Cardiovascular Dis-
    ease." *American Journal of Clinical Nutrition*, January 2010.

Willett, W. C., et al. "Intake of Trans Fatty Acids and Risk of Coronary
    Heart Disease Among Women." *Lancet* 341 (1993): 581–85.

10: SO THEN WHAT CAN YOU EAT?

Bazzano, L., et al. "Effects of Low-Carbohydrate and Low-Fat Diets:
    A Randomized Trial." *Annals of Internal Medicine* 161, no. 5 (2014):
    309–18.

Bhupathiraju, S. N. , et al. "Changes in Coffee Intake and Subsequent
    Risk of Type 2 Diabetes: Three Large Cohorts of US Men and
    Women." *Diabetologia*, April 26, 2014.

Chavarro, J. E., et al. "Soy Food and Isoflavone Intake in Relation to
    Semen Quality Parameters Among Men from an Infertility Clinic."
    Human Reproduction, 2008, doi:10.1093/humrep/den243.

Driskell, J. A., et al. "Concentrations of Selected Vitamins and Selenium
    in Bison Cuts." *Journal of Animal Science* 75 (1997): 2950.

Evert, A. B., et al. "Nutrition Therapy Recommendations for the Man-
    agement of Adults with Diabetes." *Diabetes Care* 36 (2013): 3821–42.

Fine, E. J., et al. "Targeting Insulin Inhibition as a Metabolic Therapy in
    Advanced Cancer: A Pilot Safety and Feasibility Dietary Trial in 10
    Patients." *Nutrition* 28, no. 10 (October 2012): 1028–35.

Ho, V. W., et al. "A Low Carbohydrate, High Protein Diet Slows Tumor
    Growth and Prevents Cancer Initiation." *Cancer Research* 71, no. 13
    (July 2011): 4484–93.

Ketogenic Diet Resource. www.ketogenic-diet-resource/ketoacidosis
    .html.

Krebs-Smith, Susan M., Patricia M. Guenther, Amy F. Subar, Sharon I.

Kirkpatrick, and Kevin W. Dodd. "Americans Do Not Meet Federal Dietary Recommendations." *Journal of Nutrition* 140 (2010): 1832–38.

Marchello, M. J., et al. "Nutrient Composition of Bison Fed Concentrate Diets." *Journal of Food Composition and Analysis* 11 (1998): 231.

Mercola, Dr. Joseph. "The Health Dangers of Soy." *Huffington Post*, August 23, 2012, http://www.huffingtonpost.com/dr-mercola/soy-health_b_1822466.html.

Mohammed, G. Abdelwahab, et al. "The Ketogenic Diet Is an Effective Adjuvant to Radiation Therapy for the Treatment of Malignant Glioma." *PLoS ONE* 7, no. 5 (2012): e36197, doi:10.1371/journal .pone.0036197.

"Otto Warburg. Biographical." Nobelprize.org, accessed November 27, 2014.

"The Root Cause of Cancer." www.ganodermareview.com.

Sigurdsson, Axel, M.D. "Ketosis." *Doc's Opinion*, June 2, 2014, www .docsopinion.com/2014/06/02/ketosis.

Smith, Jeffrey M. "Can Genetically-Engineered Foods Explain the Exploding Gluten Sensitivity?" *Institute for Responsible Technology*, 2013.

Telchoiz, Nancy. "What if Bad Fat Is Actually Good for You?" *Men's Health*, October 10, 2007.

Thomson, Julie. "Graham Crackers Were Invented to Curb Your Sexual Desires." *Huffington Post*, June 8, 2014, http://www.huffingtonpost .com/2014/08/08/graham-cracker-history-sexual-urges_n_5629961 .html.

Wagh, K., et al. "Lactose Persistence and Lipid Pathway Selection in the Maasai." *PloS ONE* 7, no. 9 (2012): e44751, doi:10,1371/journal.pone .0044751.

Willett, Walter C., M.D., et al. "Coffee Consumption and Coronary Heart Disease in Women." *JAMA* 275, no. 6 (1996): 458–62, doi:10.1001/ jama, 1996.03530300042038.

INDEX

Page numbers in *italic* refer to illustrations.

ABOUT THE AUTHORS

―――――――

DR. RICHARD P. JACOBY is one of the country's leading peripheral nerve surgeons. He practices in Scottsdale, Arizona, and specializes in the treatment of peripheral neuropathy. He is one of the co-founders of the Scottsdale Healthcare Wound Management Center and is the past president of the Arizona Podiatry Association and the Association of Extremity Nerve Surgeons. He is a diplomate of the American Board of Podiatric Surgery and is a member of the American Podiatry Association, the Arizona Podiatry Association, and the Association of Extremity Nerve Surgeons. He lives in Scottsdale with his wife and two children.

RAQUEL BALDELOMAR is the founder of Quaintise, a health care marketing and advertising agency. An expert in medical marketing strategies, she helps organizations transform sick care into true health care. She is a contributing writer for *Advertising Age*, *Modern Healthcare*, and *Physician* magazine and is a reporter on how digital health and wireless technology empower consumers to take control of their own health. She lives in Santa Monica, California.